the **complete flier's** handbook

Brian Clegg is a Cambridge science graduate who worked
for British Airways for seventeen years, managing development in many aspects of the airline business from scheduling
and yield management to baggage handling and check-in.
In 1994 he left BA to set up his own business, and he now
advises a wide range of clients on business creativity and
customer services. He is also a freelance journalist and the
author of a number of books, most recently *Light Years*, an
exploration of humanity's fascination with light.

He lives in Wiltshire with his wife and two children.

the **complete flier's** handbook

the essential guide to
successful air travel

BRIAN CLEGG

Pan Books

First published 2002 by Pan
an imprint of Pan Macmillan Ltd
Pan Macmillan, 20 New Wharf Road, London N1 9RR
Basingstoke and Oxford
Associated companies throughout the world
www.panmacmillan.com

ISBN 0330 48917 8

A CIP catalogue record for this book is available from
the British Library.

Typeset by SetSystems Ltd, Saffron, Walden, Essex
Printed and bound in Great Britain by
Mackays of Chatham plc, Chatham, Kent

Contents

contents

Acknowledgements

Many thanks to my agent, Peter Cox, for prodding me into action, and to Catherine Whitaker and her colleagues at Macmillan for making it a pleasure to write. A particular thank you to Jerry Schemmel for permission to reproduce a section from his book *Chosen To Live* (Victory Publishing Company, Littleton, Co., USA).

Thanks also to the many people who have provided me with travellers' tales and tips, including Liz Bates, Pam Beckley, Paul Birch, Peggy Brusseau, Kevin Coleman, Todd Curtis, Stewart Desson, Diana Fairechild, David Freemantle, Nick Gassman, Gary Gray, Andy and Fiona Grüneberg, Helmut Jakubowicz, Sarah James, Farrol Kahn, Vasko Kohlmayer, Ken Lowe, Brian Martin and Jayne Spooner.

Introduction

Air passengers should get more information about the health risks of flying . . . Our concern is not that health is secondary to safety but that it has been woefully neglected.

House of Lords Science and Technology Committee,
Wednesday 22 November 2000

Air travel is a relatively new addition to human capabilities. There are still people alive who were born before the achievement of powered flight. Commercial air travel has passed through a number of phases in its lifetime. Initially it was regarded as racy, as a mode of transport suited only to those who were prepared to take their lives into their hands. Later it became seen as opulent and luxurious, the privilege of the jet set. But towards the end of the twentieth century air travel had become so common that it was regarded as just another everyday form of transport.

The latest change in image in some ways returns air travel to its earliest days. As we have learned more about the dangers of being in such a hostile environment as an aircraft cabin, air travellers have been thinking more and more about the health risks they are facing, treating a plane trip as they would a stay in hospital – an unfortunate but necessary spell in an unhealthy location. The terrible events of 11 September 2001, culminating in the destruction of four passenger aircraft and the World Trade Center in New York add to this tension.

There is no doubt that there is cause for concern, that the environment on board an aircraft is one that we need to be prepared to counter. But there is no reason why the experience of flying has to be a bad one. As long, for instance, as we are aware that security is necessary to avoid another terrorist atrocity, it need not be an irritant. Now we know that exposure to the sun's rays is bad for us we take the appropriate precautions, but still enjoy our holidays. Similarly, knowledge of the dangers of flight should not put us off air travel, but merely encourage us to make sure that we are suitably prepared.

Despite my seventeen years in the airline industry, I used to be a nervous flier. This was not because of a lack of experience, or of technical knowledge of how aircraft operated. I finally discovered that for me, with a background in statistics, the real problem was a lack of trust in the glib assurance that 'It's safer to travel by air than by car.' By getting to grips with what the airline safety statistics really mean, I was able for the first time to fully understand just how safe flying really is.

Similarly, my intention is not to turn you, the reader, into a nervous wreck, but to give you the information that you need to make the best of the air-travel experience – to thrive on flying. Whether you need to know how to make the most of your air ticket or what to do if your baggage is damaged, having the right information can make all the difference. And by putting the risks into perspective, having discovered the reality of the statistics of air safety that always seem to conceal as much as they reveal, it is possible to make intelligent judgements on when and how to make use of the plane.

After all, there is no doubt that, both for business and pleasure, the ability to fly the world has transformed our lives. I hope that this book will help to make flying a more straightforward and a more pleasurable experience.

→ Fast Track: Getting Started

This book is designed either to be read through or to be dipped into when you have a specific requirement. Here are a few starting points:

- Need to choose the right ticket? p. 6

- Want to be sure you have made all the right preparations? p. 31

- Want to get the best seat at check-in? p. 72

- Worried about deep-vein thrombosis? p. 90

- Unhappy with aircraft air? p. 102 & 117

- Concerned about radiation exposure at altitude? p. 132

- Want to deal with jet lag? p. 144

- Stressed out by flying? p. 160

- Or downright scared? p. 176

- Want to make the most of your time on board? p. 183

- Terrified at the thought of flying with kids? p. 202

- Do you have special physical needs? p. 225

- Is your pet travelling? p. 238

- Lost your bags? p. 247

- Been bumped or delayed? p. 254

- Want to know how safe it *really* is to fly? p. 260

- What is it like to be in a plane crash? p. 280

- Where can you get online information? p. 323

- What's the airport code for your destination? p. 341

- Worried about hotel safety? p. 398

1 Choosing Your Flight

In the chapters that follow we will cover the whole experience of flight, exploring ways to survive and thrive on air travel. It all begins with the ticket.

Purchasing an airline ticket isn't like going out and choosing a new car or shopping for groceries. You are buying something intangible: the ability to move from one part of the world to another, combined with the experience, good or bad, of being in an aircraft. You are buying a unique mix of allure, fear, inconvenience, excitement and irritation, when all you really want to do is get from A to B.

It is common these days to proclaim the death of the glamour of flying. I'd dispute that. Flying certainly isn't the same experience that we had twenty years ago. There are many more people crammed into the planes and airports. Expectations are higher than ever before. But, even so, some of the fascination remains. Compare the atmosphere at an airport, a bus station and a railway station. The frisson of danger accompanying flight combined with all those exotic-sounding destinations keeps an element of opulent excitement in place however much the commentators like to say it has been lost.

The price that won't stay fixed

The whole process starts well before you reach the bustle of the airport, though. The choices to be made begin with the purchase of the ticket – an apparently simple consideration that is, in fact, frighteningly complex. This reflects the unusual nature of airline inventory. A manufacturer's stock may gradually decline in value, but airline seats have a much more complex history, varying in price with time, from the moment they are first loaded on to the reservation system to minutes before take-off. Once the plane pushes back from the stand, the value of an empty seat finally and irrevocably drops to nothing.

It's the economics of running an airline that dictates the fluctuations in price. A number of full-fare seats are held back because business travellers may want to book at the last minute, and so are prepared to pay a premium. The airline wants to make sure that there are enough seats left for these high-paying customers. But it also wants to sell the rest of the seats. These are therefore made available earlier on, from when the flight is entered into the reservations computer, as far ahead as a year before departure day. To make early booking more attractive, some seats carry lower pricing in those early months.

Ideally (from the airline's viewpoint) every plane would depart full. It would have the maximum number of high-fare-paying business passengers, and every other seat would be filled with the less lucrative leisure passengers. Of course reality is rarely like this. The number of seats blocked off for the late bookers can never be more than a guess, based on history. If there aren't enough seats, the flight is liable to be overbooked (see page 67). If too many seats are held back, the flight will leave half empty – unless it can be filled with standby passengers.

The great era of standby is now over. The theory was that it was worth getting some money – any money – out of those otherwise empty seats. By waiting until a few minutes before departure, standby passengers could snap up any leftover seats for a fraction of the usual fare. But this scheme overlooked the costs of keeping the passengers fed and watered on board, and the inconvenience of disrupting carefully calculated catering numbers. Few airlines now sell standby tickets – most standby travellers are airline employees – but they are occasionally still available. You may also be offered standby if you arrive at the airport early and want to try for an earlier flight, or if you miss your flight and want to go for a later one.

So what should the traveller choose? From personal experience, I wouldn't recommend trying standby (in the rare cases that it is available) unless you are young and fancy-free. If you can cope with not knowing exactly when you are going to leave, and don't mind last-minute changes of plan, it's fine. Otherwise the nerve-tingling wait at the gate will simply pile on the pressure in what is already a stressful situation. There can be few more painful moments than when you are about to be accepted to travel and suddenly the lost passenger that you have been praying wouldn't arrive comes haring up to the gate and you know that you are off the flight and have to rethink your journey. It simply isn't worth the hassle.

→ Fast Track: Deciding on Your Ticketing Strategy

Have a clear idea of your budget and requirements before looking for a suitable fare.

- If you are going to a business meeting, find out the address and obtain an estimate of the driving time from the airport to that address before making your booking.

- If you are attending an organized event, check the details for required arrival and departure times – you may have to make sure your booking matches them.

- If you are travelling near a public holiday (at either end of the flight), watch out for price hikes – see if you can avoid the peak times and premium fares.

- By staying over a Saturday night, you may be able to save sufficient money on a fare to pay the hotel bill for your extra stay.

- If you are travelling in a group (typically ten or more), you should be able to get a discount. Don't be afraid to ask.

- If you are booking several itineraries through different agents, make sure you don't accidentally book yourself twice on the same flight. Airlines have automated systems that may cancel both bookings if you do.

Taking the long view

If an early booking suits you, it is possible to make considerable savings with none of the on-the-day stress of standby. These savings are offered to try to fill the seats that won't be taken by high-paying business people, and to obtain them you are likely to have to book well in advance. It also helps to avoid travelling in business hours, and you may have to commit to staying over a weekend.

These advance-booking offers are known as saver or excursion fares, or more grandly as advance-purchase excursion – APEX for short. If you want a cheap flight, bear in mind that the more flexible you can be (not, for example, specifying exact dates), the better the chances of coming up with a particularly low fare.

Airlines are generally smart businesses, making sure that as much as possible of the risk of accepting a long-term booking is transferred to the customer. Whereas an unused full-fare, late-booked ticket can be cashed in at any time, even after the flight, APEX tickets and their equivalents are usually not refundable and can't be transferred to someone else. What's more, sometimes you can't even change a detail, and if you can there is likely to be an administrative charge. There's no such thing as a free lunch – or a cheap ticket without plenty of restrictions.

Often the cheap tickets will sell out very quickly, but this doesn't mean that it's impossible to pick up a bargain weeks after the tickets are first released. Some airlines, for example, release seats over time. If you don't get anything straight away, keep trying. It's worth finding out when the advance-purchase deadline is, because quite often seats are made available shortly before that deadline.

Note, by the way, if you intend to make use of such cheap fares, that there is a particularly bizarre aspect of the pricing. An APEX return trip is often cheaper than a single ticket (which is pretty well always full price). For a one-way trip, this makes it cost-effective to buy a return ticket and simply not use the second part. The airlines are not amused by this practice, but there isn't a lot they can do about it.

Similarly, if you want to avoid the restrictions of 'including a weekend' or a minimum stay that are usually imposed with APEX, you still might save money by buying two overlapping APEX return tickets rather than going for a full-fare short-stay ticket. Watch out though – when you don't turn up for the outbound leg of your second ticket, the airline may cancel the whole thing. Contact airline reservations and let them know you can't make that flight, but will still be returning, so that they can protect the return leg. These savings aren't guaranteed – always check the pricing.

Other saving tips

It isn't just by buying in advance that you can cut the cost of flying. It's worth shopping around – airlines' prices are not all the same at any one time. It's also worth thinking about your airports. If you are travelling to or from a large city there may well be a choice. Going for one of the less popular points of departure or entry can save cash. If you are travelling from London, for example, don't assume that Heathrow is the only option. From New York you have the choice of JFK, La Guardia and Newark.

Some airlines are more equal than others

The range of ticket types available can be bewildering, but you will also need to pick an airline. Again, if you want to keep the cost down you can't afford to be fussy. With special offers, limited-applicability deals and all the marketing paraphernalia available to the modern airline, the cheapest option will vary from day to day. If you have a preference for a particular carrier, you have to be prepared to pay a little extra to make sure you get that choice.

Before you do express a preference, think a little about the criteria you might have for choosing an airline. Make sure that the decisive factor is not advertising. Airline companies are past masters at selling on image, at giving you a soft-focus, pastel-coloured impression of comfort and service. Instead, try to use more objective measures. One might be safety (see page 310 for a comparison of airlines' safety). Another might be a more realistic assessment of what the airline's facilities and staff are like – talk to other customers about their experience.

Also, you might consider what you are looking for in a flight. Some airlines sell their product on being exotic and unusual, but this might not be what you want while ten kilometres up in the air. Instead it could be much better to have reassurance and familiarity. There's a lot to be said in this respect for flying with an airline whose first language is the same as your own.

→ Fast Track:
Questions to Ask the Ticket Agent

- Will the fare be different if I fly on a different day, or a different flight, or if I stay away a Saturday night, or if I book further in advance?

- Is this a confirmed reservation?

- Will I be able to change my reservation?

- Will I be charged for doing so?

- Will I get my money back if I cancel?

- Are there any other restrictions on this fare?

- Is this a non-stop flight?

- Is this a non-smoking flight?

- Can the airline accommodate my special needs?

- What is my baggage allowance?

Making the deal

So you have decided on your type of ticket; now you have to purchase it. Until recently the choices came down to popping into a travel agent or ringing an airline direct, but the Web has opened up a whole range of new options, with direct ticketing from most airlines and a variety of operators offering cheap tickets to a wide choice of destinations.

Quick Tip: **Paper or E-Ticket**

Traditional tickets come as a long rectangular slip of paper with a voucher for each leg of your journey. Increasingly, though, airlines are making use of e-tickets, where you are issued with only a booking reference code. If you opt for an e-ticket, make sure that your airline or agent provides you with a detailed itinerary, showing such information as your booking reference, your flight numbers, the departure and arrival times, and the meal codes (see page 234). It's a good idea to get such an itinerary even if you have a paper ticket – it's easier to read, and you can leave a copy at home so you are easier to contact.

When you arrive at the airport with an e-ticket, make sure you have both your printed itinerary and your e-ticket receipt with you. Take your passport as well, even if you are flying domestically, as you will need to prove your identity.

If your time is valuable, you are still best advised to go to a reputable travel agent and let experience with the computer terminal win you a good price. (If it becomes obvious that the agent is having trouble with the computer system, it pays to go elsewhere. These systems require expertise to get the best out of them, and agents are going to miss opportunities if they don't know exactly what they are doing.) Using an agent has the advantage both of saving time up front and also that it should be easier to make a change later on with an agent to help.

Quick Tip: Advance and be Recognized

Frequent-flier schemes (see page 22) are used to encourage loyalty – but there's something else in them for you. If you are loyal to a particular travel agent or airline, it will begin to recognize you, either directly or through its computer system. And recognition means that it is more likely to do you a favour and more likely to match your requirements every time.

If you would rather invest some of your time to have more control, try using the Web. Check the pricing on airlines' web sites (see page 323). Then try out some of the cheap-ticket vendors. Bear in mind, though, that these often show only a minimum price for a route. When you give the system all the details of when you want to travel, you will find with irritating regularity that you are informed that there are no bookings available. Still, with patience you should be able to find yourself a bargain. There is the usual buyer's caveat when using the Web – make sure you are dealing with a reputable, traceable company before giving it your credit-card details. In particular, make sure there are valid 'real-world' contact details (phone, address, fax). I am always very suspicious of companies that can't be contacted any other way than through their web sites.

These cheap-flight web sites are modern versions of the bucket shop – companies specializing in buying up unwanted seats cheaply and selling them on. Traditional bucket shops still exist – look out for advertisements in newspapers and on Teletext – and, like the cheap web sites, these can really save money if you don't need to be sure until fairly late in the day exactly when you will travel. Make sure you know exactly what you are buying, though. For example, a bucket shop may well be selling seats on an under-filled charter flight. This will have a different (even lower than usual) class of catering and less legroom than a scheduled flight.

One point is essential with international flights: make sure at the time your ticket is issued that the name on it matches the name in your passport. Book a ticket in the exact form your name has in the passport. The airline may accept a ticket for Dave Smith if your passport says David Smith, but there's no guarantee that it will. This is particularly important if you use a nickname or if your name is shortened in an unusual way – I have seen a passenger have to buy a new ticket because an airline would not accept that Kit was short for Christopher. If you have recently changed your name (for instance, through getting married), make sure you have appropriate documentation to prove that you are who you say you are.

If the agent makes a mistake it can easily be corrected on the spot. If you don't realize until later, you may be charged for the issuing of a new ticket (as the name usually can't be changed). Obviously, with a ticket coming through the mail your first chance of making this check is when the ticket arrives. Again, the issuer should be prepared to correct mistakes at this point.

Quick Tip: Take Note

By keeping note of a couple of essentials you can minimize the risk of pain further down the line. Always keep your confirmation document or the ticket number ('record locator' or 'booking identifier' – usually a sequence of letters) handy in case changes need to be made.

When you make the initial reservation, and particularly if you make any subsequent changes, always make a note of the person you talked to, and when. If any problems arise you will be able to refer back to this transaction.

When you get your ticket, also check that the little box that says 'Status' contains the word 'OK'. This shows that your reservation is confirmed. If anything else is in that box it's worth checking just what is going on.

If you aren't picking up your ticket on the spot, get the airline or agent to fax a confirmation of your reservation. It will be useful if there are any problems when you arrive at the airport, and will help back up subsequent claims if things go wrong.

✔ Checklist: Ticket Check
A few quick points to check on receiving your ticket

- ❑ Name exactly matches name on passport
- ❑ Correct destination
- ❑ Correct flight
- ❑ Correct dates
- ❑ Correct class
- ❑ Correct meal code (see page 234 for the codes used)
- ❑ Status box shows 'OK'

Pick a route, any route

As if there isn't enough complexity in choosing an airline and a ticket, another potential variable is the route to get to your destination. At one time there was little choice – you flew with your country's flag carrier, the airline given special access to the routes out of your country, or you used its opposite number from your destination. Though the airline world has not been totally deregulated (realistically, this will never happen, as the number of slots available for aircraft to take off and land in at popular airports like

London's Heathrow will always limit how many airlines can operate), things are much less simple now.

I was speaking the other day to a regular traveller who works for the British office of a German bank. He pointed out that, rather than fly direct from London to Tokyo, his bank expected him to fly via Frankfurt, because the resultant pair of flights cost less than the single non-stop flight. It is certainly worth costing some obvious alternative routes through nearby major airports, but be careful when doing so that you put all the elements into the equation – the decision isn't all about cost.

In this particular instance, my informant's bank was saving around £500 by taking this measure. As we will see in a moment, this may have been worthwhile. But the accountants were also recommending making a similar diversion via Frankfurt when travelling from London to New York. Let's look at what should have gone into the balance there.

On the plus side, the diversion via Frankfurt would have saved between £50 and £100 on the London to New York fare. But to achieve it the flier had to travel in almost the opposite direction, increasing the overall journey distance by around 1,200 km. From a safety viewpoint, the number of take-offs and landings the flier went through was doubled, and, as these are the most dangerous parts of the flight, his risk was also increased.

In more quantifiable terms, the overall round-trip journey time was pushed up from around 14 hours to 20 hours. That was rating the traveller's time as low as £10 an hour – not much for an employee of a merchant bank. If the passenger had baggage, there was also an increased risk of losing the bags as they passed through yet another baggage system. Overall, the costs that were undergone to save a meagre amount of money simply did not justify the action.

Let's look again at the Tokyo trip. When I checked out the straight fares it turned out that there was hardly any saving at all by changing at Frankfurt, but the round-trip flying time went up from twenty-four hours to thirty-two That is eight extra hours of inconvenience to pay for. Accepting that the bank in question might have had a special deal with a German airline, even £500 might be considered doubtful compensation for wasting a useful day and decreasing the effectiveness of the traveller after a more stressful and unsettled journey.

Sometimes, of course, you can find real bargains. When researching the options, I found a special rate that saved over £700 on the standard fare. Worthwhile at last? Maybe not. This special rate required a change in Singapore and a total round-trip journey time of a staggering fifty hours. Of course if you are travelling on a tight budget it might be worth such delays and the extra stress to save money. And it may be that you want a stopover at an intermediate destination. But for many business travellers it's just not worth introducing a secondary destination to cut costs.

What is direct?

At least in such circumstances the decision to take a stopover is conscious, but it is less than funny if the airline imposes an extra landing without you even realizing that it is going to happen. This is entirely possible, thanks to the misleading terms that are traditional in the airline world. It would be reasonable to assume that a direct flight takes you straight from A to B. In fact it can just as easily take you from A to F to X to B. This is particularly likely to happen when travelling to a relatively obscure US destination or when flying through tightly grouped smaller cities – for example, around the Caribbean. As long as the same plane is used to get you from A to B it is, in airline terms, a direct flight, even if you have to get off the plane at one or more intermediate stops. What you were probably hoping for was a non-stop flight – this genuinely does get you from A to B without any landings in between.

Less misleading is the concept of a connecting flight. At least the name does make it clear that there is a need to transfer to another plane en route – to make a connection. This term is used in Europe to mean both connections within an airline and connections to other airlines' flights. For example, if you fly into London Heathrow on Cathay Pacific, you might have a connection on to a British Airways internal flight to Glasgow. In the USA, however, a connecting flight is sometimes more tightly defined as being a flight that links to another plane of the same airline. If this is the case, a transfer to another airline is called a through flight – again a confusing label that doesn't really indicate what is involved.

If you have to suffer a transit stop, try to make use of it. Transit lounges are dismal places. Look for an opportunity to do something more than sit in one of those serried rows of seats. As long as you have appropriate documentation (passport, ticket, boarding pass) you may (no guarantees) be able to get out into the airport proper. If you do, though, make sure you have a cast-iron way of keeping track of the time. A transit airport is not a place in which to be left behind.

Early pickings

Although most people still have their seat allocated at check-in, it is possible to specify a seat before the departure day, once the flight has been loaded into the departure-control computer (this takes place between a month and ninety days before the flight). See page 72 for advice on selecting a seat, but those who want to get an early seat allocation will have to be aware of just what the significance of the various seat numbers is. Luckily, many airlines now feature seat plans of the aircraft on their web sites, and you can find out if 8C really is an aisle seat on the upper deck. Appendix 5 (page 323) contains pointers to many of the airlines' sites.

Late bookers may be able to get a seat allocated at the time of purchase. Alternatively, a small number of airlines now provide the ability to check in online the night before. For example, holders of the British Airways silver and gold club cards can check in and choose a seat online between twenty-four hours before the flight and the final hour or two. You may also find some downtown check-in sites. London's Paddington station, for example, with its fifteen-minute fast trains to Heathrow, has check-in facilities complete with baggage collection for all the major airlines. Such facilities were suspended after the New York tragedy in September 2001, but may now be reinstated.

Piling up the miles

Like most large businesses, airlines are interested in knowing all they can about their passengers, and in getting them to return time and again. The two weapons that the airlines use are frequent-flier programmes, in which miles travelled are added up to provide future benefits like free leisure tickets, and executive clubs, which provide special privileges to the regular flier. Usually the two are combined into a single scheme.

In theory, the frequent-flier programmes are designed to lock you into using a particular airline to accumulate miles, but in practice many of the schemes are linked in complex networks of alliances and partnerships that make it possible to combine miles from different airlines to build up impressive allocations even if you don't stick to the same carrier. For example the One World alliance (see below) allows frequent-flier miles to be combined in a single system. There are also usually interchanges of points outside the system, so, for example, British Airways points can be accumulated from Alaska Airlines, America West, Emirates, JAL and LOT as well as from the One World carriers. Similar schemes exist among other airlines as the Star, Skyteam and Wings alliances.

→ Fast Track:
The Alliances

The frequent-flier alliances change regularly – see the web sites on page 325 for up-to-date memberships. At the time of writing the big three were:

- One World – Aer Lingus, American Airlines, British Airways, Cathay Pacific, Finnair, Iberia, LanChile and Qantas

- Skyteam – Aeromexico, Air France, CSA Czech Airlines, Delta and Korean

- Star – Air Canada, Air New Zealand, ANA, Ansett Australia, Austrian, British Midland, Lauda Air, Lufthansa, Mexicana, SAS, Singapore Airlines, Thai, Tyrolean, United and Varig.

with KLM and Northwest making up a fourth which was intended to be called Wings, but now seems to be simply 'the Northwest KLM alliance'.

Airlines both inside and outside alliances also have one-to-one partnerships with other airlines for exchanging points. Check the airline's customer-services department or web site for details.

The exact meaning of these mileage-based schemes can be unclear, particularly when combined with the independent offering (originally set up by British Airways) Air Miles. Air Miles are available from a number of non-airline sources, such as the Sainsbury's supermarket loyalty card, and convert fairly literally to miles of travel. By comparison, the miles accumulated on an airline's frequent-flier scheme may well be miles flown, and many more are required to travel the same nominal distance.

Frequent-flier schemes are worth pursuing, but bear in mind the restrictions that will be placed on the free tickets you can take up as a result of your accumulated points. These may limit you to certain times of the day or days of the week, and there will also be all-out forbidden periods – for example, around Thanksgiving in the USA. Often the schemes are complex and are regularly changed – if you have a significant accumulation of frequent-flier miles it's well worth getting acquainted with the web site Points.com (see page 327), which not only has a mass of information on the different schemes but also provides an exchange facility to convert one type of points into another.

→ Fast Track:
Getting the Most out of Frequent-Flier Schemes

- If you haven't already done so, make sure you enrol with at least one member each of the One World Alliance (e.g. British Airways or American Airlines), the Star Alliance (e.g. British Midland or United), Skyteam (e.g. Air France or Delta) and the Northwest KLM alliance. You might add the other big US carriers, Southwest, US Airways and Continental. This means that, should you be moved to another airline owing to a delay or a cancellation, you will still pick up the points.

- Look out for opportunities to get bonus miles when you first sign up.

- Make sure you are a member of the appropriate scheme before making a reservation.

- If someone else is booking for you, don't be shy about giving your frequent-flier number to accompany the booking.

- Loyalty wins you extra points and 'club' benefits – if you travel regularly, try to keep your preferred carriers down to a minimum number.

- Always use your frequent-flier number when booking – it's not just for the points: you will also get better seats on heavily booked flights.

- Check for other opportunities (credit cards, hotels, hire cars etc.) to add to your frequent-flier miles.

- Have your frequent-flier ID or number with you when you check in.

Going clubbing

Executive clubs (that's the British Airways name – each airline will have its own fancy label) are an associated way to reward the regular traveller. They normally feature several different tiers, each with additional benefits, and are linked to the frequent-flier scheme, using miles accumulated to generate the membership level.

As an example, let's examine the BA scheme in a little more detail. There are four levels. Which level you are in will depend on the points you have accumulated in the last twelve months in the frequent-flier scheme. The first level – blue – has very little going for it other than being a stepping stone to the next levels up. There will be some discounts available (such as on car hire, telephone systems and hotels), and regular communication from the airline, which will record your preferences (such as seating) and try to use these when you are booking on a new flight.

Quick Tip: **Clubbing USA**

There is some evidence that it is better to join a club like the BA Executive Club from the USA rather than the UK. Because there is more competition in the USA there tend to be better privileges at any particular level, and it is easier to get moved up a level. All you need is a US address to list in your registration.

Silver is the first serious level, with automatic access to airline lounges – a very valuable asset when travelling a long distance (see page 85) that can also be accessed by travelling business class or first class. Gold adds extra lounges and the use of arrivals lounges. Premier (which used to be called platinum, but that looked too much like the plebeian silver) works rather differently from the other levels. Whereas blue, silver and gold cards are earned automatically by spending a certain amount with the company, premier membership is provided only by invitation to individuals whom the airline particularly wants to get on its side. In fact you won't even see these premier cards mentioned in the airline's marketing – it's as exclusive as that. Premier members are personally handled each time they fly, with a specialist customer-support agent who knows their preferences always on hand.

→ Fast Track:
Which Scheme to Use?

Each of the airlines' schemes has a complex, shifting mixture of pros and cons. Check the Inside Flier and Points.com web sites (see page 327) for up-to-date comparisons. Here are some key points to consider:

- What are the airport benefits offered?

- What is available online? Can you redeem immediately on-line?

- What restrictions apply?

- Do the miles and points expire?

- What executive/elite options are available? For example, some schemes make you a permanent top-level member after flying a certain number of miles.

- Are there any spouse/partner benefits?

- What upgrade options are available?

- How well does the scheme integrate with the schemes of alliance partners?

- What range of alliance partners is available?

- How are children treated? Up to what age do they get child benefits?

Ready for take-off?

Getting your booking sorted is an essential preparation, but it's not all that can be done in advance to make sure that your flight runs as smoothly as possible. The next chapter examines the preparations that can make all the difference.

✈ *Summary:* Choosing Your Flight

- Shop around to get the best deal.

- Book early if you can.

- Consider using a less popular airport.

- Check your ticket.

- Confirm your reservation.

- Select an airline on realistic criteria.

- Consider indirect routes to save money, but remember the hidden costs and the extra risk involved.

- Choose your favourite seat ahead of time.

- Join a range of frequent-flier schemes, and always register your membership when booking.

2 Be Prepared

At one time flying anywhere would have been such an upheaval that the thought of it would necessarily have been accompanied by careful preparation. Now, flying is such an everyday part of life that it is easy to underestimate what will be required. Just because it is simple to get across the world doesn't mean that you don't need to be well prepared if you are going to make your journey safely and effectively. Your pre-flight checks needn't take up much time, but it is essential that you get them in early enough.

Are you sure how far in advance you need to have a hepatitis-A injection? How long will it take you to get a visa (if you need one at all)? What should you pack, and where? It is easy to make a mistake that will spoil your whole trip. If you have a journey imminent, take a glance through the checklist below and make sure that you haven't missed anything. If you have more time, use the list as part of your preparation. A checklist isn't the sign of being an amateur traveller: it's a practical essential.

✔ Checklist: Pre-Flight Checks

Each item is discussed in more detail below, but here's a quick summary:

- ❏ Immunization up to date
- ❏ Immunization certificates obtained, if required
- ❏ E111 (medical form for European destinations) obtained
- ❏ ID – if you don't need a passport, the airline may demand other identification
- ❏ Passport valid throughout the trip
- ❏ Appropriate visas obtained
- ❏ Ticket and seating booked
- ❏ Hotel(s) booked
- ❏ Insurance arranged
- ❏ Currency arranged
- ❏ Credit cards valid throughout the trip
- ❏ Hold/hand baggage limits checked
- ❏ Political situation checked
- ❏ Transport to airport arranged
- ❏ Fully equipped (from electrical adaptors to insect repellent)

Catch the plane, nothing else

There is little joy in the contemplation of inoculations and other medical preparations for travelling, but having a certificate of inoculation is an essential to be able to travel to some countries, and for many more it is equally important for your own health that you are protected. In Appendix 1 (page 289) you will find a guide to the recommended protection for most destinations around the world at the time of writing.

It is often most straightforward to get your preventive treatment at your local doctor's surgery, but this isn't always convenient, and the surgery may not hold every vaccine in stock. If you are in a hurry, British Airways operates specialist travel clinics in the UK and South Africa (phone 01276 685040 – see page 328 for its web site), as does the Medical Advisory Service for Travellers Abroad (see page 328 for its web site), which can help out at short notice – but even the full-time travel clinics can't speed up the time a vaccination or inoculation needs to take effect, so the definition of 'last minute' is a variable commodity in this respect. Similar clinics are available throughout the USA and in major cities around the world – for example, the Overseas Travel Clinic in Battleboro, Vermont (802 258 3358) and the Healthy Traveler Clinic in Pasadena, California (626 584 1200). A worldwide list of clinics can be found on the International Society of Travel Medicine's web site (see page 328), or consult your local health organization for the nearest clinic.

As well as the injections, remember that there may be a need for other medical drugs – most commonly the controversial anti-malarial treatment. This is controversial because a number of regular travellers have suggested that the side effects of some anti-malarial treatments can be just as bad as the illness itself. You will find there is a complex balance between effectiveness and the level of possible complications.

At the time of writing, chloroquine was the recommended anti-malarial drug of choice where there isn't a resistance to it. The most common alternative, mefloquine (trade name Lariam), has had considerable doubts raised about its side effects and needs to be administered with care. In May 2001 a new product, Malarone, was licensed that is claimed to be as effective as Lariam without the side effects, though it is significantly more expensive. There are other alternatives – getting the right anti-malarial protection is a subject where you may find it useful to take specialist advice rather than relying on your GP alone. Remember that all anti-malarial drugs should continue to be taken for four weeks after the trip.

Although technically not medical, you will also need some form of insect repellent in areas where attacks by insects are common or potentially dangerous. Apart from anything else, no anti-malarial treatment is absolutely guaranteed to work, so the more you can reduce the chances of being bitten in the first place, the more likely it is that you can resist infection.

Quick Tip: **What to Get**

For an immediate update on the recommended inoculations for travelling to any country in the world, see the UK Department of Health's web site at www.doh.gov.uk/ traveladvice. Details are also provided in Appendix 1 on page 294.

Going alternative

If you are concerned about the possible side effects of medical treatments, there are homoeopathic remedies available. These can be used to overcome the side effects of immunization, or potentially to replace some immunizations, though I cannot recommend using them in this way unless it is fully supported by your doctor.

A number of reputable homoeopathic pharmacies now have web sites where you can find out more about what is available (see page 328). For simple ailments it is practical to resort to self-treatment, but for anything more I recommend using an appropriate practitioner. Although such people are few and far between, the best option is to find a qualified GP who also prescribes homoeopathic remedies, so that you can be sure of the entire range of possibilities available to you and what their all-round health implications are.

→ Fast Track:
Homoeopathic Remedies for Travellers

These are some of the recommendations made by the long-established Ainsworths pharmacy. See its web site (page 328) for more information. I cannot guarantee the effectiveness of any of these claims.

- Immediate effects of injury and trauma – arnica 30 reduces inflammation, bruising and shock, and promotes healing.

- Traveller's tummy – arsenica alba 30.

- Sunstroke, sun headaches, fevers, earache – belladonna 30.

- Jet lag – arnica 30 or cocculus 30.

- Travel sickness – cocculus 30 (needs to be taken before the journey and every four hours during the journey).

- Bites and puncture wounds – ledum 30.

- Overindulgence, effects of alcohol and rich/spicy foods – nux vomica 30.

- Food poisoning and septic fevers – pyrogen 200.

Taking it with you

If you are on medication for an existing condition, apart from the obvious requirement to take the drugs with you, make sure you that you keep your medicines in the original containers. Carry appropriate information on your person in an easily located place. If your medication involves syringes or other sharp objects contact the airline to check on procedure.

A final medical consideration is the provision of both a DIY first-aid kit and a medical kit to keep you safe where local facilities aren't up to scratch. The first-aid kit is for your own use, while the medical kit contains items that you would never use yourself but that can be made available to local medics in case of emergency. These kits might never be needed, but they are not hugely expensive and give some peace of mind. They can be bought from pharmacists and travel medical centres, or direct from the suppliers: Appendix 2 (page 308) includes a checklist of essentials to ensure that a medical support kit will deliver the necessary goods.

Fit to fly?

The human body wasn't designed for the environment inside a plane. Most of the time it simply needs to adapt, but there are medical conditions that will be aggravated by the stress, low air pressure, cramped conditions and poor seating design. No matter how well prepared you are, if you are in any doubt about your fitness to fly, check with your doctor first. The checklist below highlights a number of conditions where this is absolutely essential, but such a list can never be comprehensive – always err on the side of caution.

✔ *Checklist: See Your GP*

If you suffer from any of the following medical conditions it is essential to discuss the risk with your GP before flying. Even if your condition isn't on this list, see your GP if you are in any doubt:

❑ Alcoholic addiction – *delirium tremens or Korsakoff's syndrome*
❑ Blood disorders – *anaemia, haemophilia, leukaemia*
❑ Brain disorders – *apoplexy, tumours, epilepsy, unstabilized stroke*

❑ Cardiovascular diseases – *angina pectoris, atherosclerosis, cerebrovascular accident, congenital heart disease (with poor climatic tolerances), congestive failure, deep-vein thrombosis, severe hypertension, coronary thrombosis (myocardial infarction), unstable arrhythmia, valvular lesions*
❑ Contagious diseases
❑ Gastrointestinal diseases – *acute diverticulitis, acute gastroenteritis, acute oesophageal varices, peptic ulcer, ulcerative colitis*
❑ Large unsupported hernia
❑ Pneumothorax or pneumoperitoneum
❑ Post-surgical conditions – *unstabilized convalescent and post-operative*
❑ Progressive kidney or liver failure
❑ Recent surgery – *abdominal, chest, ear, facial (but after all surgery, ensure healing time)*
❑ Respiratory diseases – *chronic asthma, bronchiectasis, chronic bronchitis, bullous lung disease, congenital pulmonary cysts, pulmonary heart disease, emphysema, lobectomy, pneumonia, pneumonectomy, tuberculosis*
❑ Severe diabetes mellitus

If you suffer from a serious or chronic illness, the airline may require you to provide a medical information form, filled in by your GP, to help it assess whether or not you should be allowed on the plane. This is not a matter of discrimination – it is in neither your interest nor the airline's if you become severely ill or die in mid-flight.

As with all bureaucratic preparations, allow plenty of time to get the form processed. If you don't have much time you will have to go direct to the airline's medics. Bear in mind, though, that the airline may respond to your form by saying no, you can't fly. Or it may insist that you will have to pay for supplementary oxygen.

If you need such certification, be aware of the statistics. The fact is that a much higher number of form-holders develop medical problems on board or soon after arrival than do ordinary travellers. The acceptance of your form does not show that you are perfectly safe to fly, just that the airline is prepared to accept the risk. It may be that you would be better to put off your flight or look for another way to travel.

Permission to enter

Check that your passport is valid well in advance – it can take a considerable time to get a new one. Make sure too that it will remain valid throughout your stay abroad, covering any possible extensions to your visit that might happen intentionally or accidentally. If you need to replace a passport quickly, many countries now have a fast-track system where you pay a little more and get a guaranteed speed of response. In the UK this is most conveniently available through the Post Office, and cuts down the delay to a fraction of the usual waiting time. UK passports are processed in this way in two weeks for a 15 per cent surcharge on the price.

UK travellers needing a passport in less than two weeks will have to go direct to a passport office. This can involve a whole day's waiting, and will incur a surcharge of 50 per cent. In a genuine emergency, the Passport Agency will deal with an application for travel in less than forty-eight hours – though it is sensible to ring the Agency first to make sure you have all appropriate documentation. The UK Passport Office is currently trialling an online application – see its web site (page 327) for details. For other countries, consult your government web site as a starting point, or the ministry dealing with internal affairs.

Visa stipulations come and go, hence the need to check well in advance for requirements. When I first began transatlantic flying I needed a visa to enter the USA – something that now seems bizarre. But don't make the mistake of thinking that a visa is something that you can get away without, or that can be arranged at the last minute. Unless it makes a mistake, the airline won't even let you travel without the appropriate visa, as it will be fined heavily for carrying you if you do.

Some visas, particularly those for ex-Communist-bloc countries, take a lot of arranging. Check with your government's travel-advice unit (in the UK, the Foreign and Commonwealth Travel Advice Unit, 020 7008 0232; in the USA, the State Department Travel Unit, 202 663 1225 – see page 327 for web sites) to ensure that you have what's needed.

Carrying cash

There is less need to arrange foreign cash in advance than was once the case. It's a good idea to have some available for immediate purchases (say a day's worth), but generally you can do just as well on the spot with your credit cards and bank cards, using traveller's cheques as back-up. If you can't get local currency and want some back-up cash, the best worldwide option is US dollars.

When you are getting currency abroad, bear in mind that exchange rates will vary from location to location. The best rates will usually come from an ATM (a cash machine) or a bank, with bureaux de change rather worse, and hotels charging even more. Don't be tempted to go for black-market exchange, however tempting the rates may seem – some countries treat this as a serious crime, and you will be an easy target for fraud.

Although it is less common than it once was, some countries still impose exchange controls, limiting the amount of foreign currency that you can take into the country or of local currency that can be taken out with you. Several of the travel-information sites listed in Appendix 5 (page 326) give information on the limitations that are currently in place.

It's in the bag

Packing is mostly a matter of common sense, but there are some special requirements for the air traveller to consider.

Quick Tip: Desert Island Essential

A scientist friend who spends much of his life jetting from conference to conference recommends one item in the luggage above all others: 'Always carry a short-wave radio. I have a cigarette-packet-sized Sony, which would definitely be my luxury item for a desert island. An amplifying antenna is also invaluable when going to really remote places.' The ability to keep in touch with the familiar world wherever you are, and to have instant entertainment in your pocket, is very attractive. Bear in mind, though, that radios should never be used on board aircraft (see page 196).

The secret of packing for air travel is not so much the quality of your folding, but how much you can get into a carry-on bag. There is a huge advantage to avoiding the hold altogether. You will miss out on the seemingly interminable wait at the baggage carousels, where inevitably your bags come out last. And you won't have the experience of a colleague who recently arrived back from a trip to find the remains of his luggage on the carousel in taped-up plastic bags. His suitcase had been destroyed in a mysterious accident, and much of his belongings had been lost with it.

Don't assume, though, that you will get away with anything in the cabin. Although some airlines allow suit carriers (particularly in first class, where there is a fair amount of wardrobe space), you are usually restricted to bags that can be placed under the seat in front of you or in the overhead lockers. Before packing, check with your airline how big a bag you can get on board. Ask too for the maximum weight and the maximum number of pieces. Many airlines restricted hand baggage to one item, counting even a handbag (purse) after the World Trade Center disaster, but some may now allow more.

→ Fast Track:
  Packing

Make a quick list of what you pack, and carry it with you in case you need to claim for lost baggage.

• Clothing – visualize your trip day by day, so that you take appropriate numbers of garments.

• Medication – make sure you take enough, that you keep it in the original containers with any documentation, and that it is accessible on the aircraft.

• Shoes – keep to a minimum: they're heavy. Pack them in a

carrier bag, so that they can be repacked dirty without messing up the rest of your luggage.

• Suits – however good you are at packing, these always get creased. Use a suit carrier if the airline will allow it on board.

• Toiletries – keep in a small soap bag, easily accessible in your hand luggage, to use them on board if necessary.

• No sharps – avoid all sharp objects including nail scissors and needles. These will be confiscated.

Size restrictions vary a little between airlines, but often the limits are 60 cm by 45 by 22. Technically there is a weight limit – between 6 and 18 kg, depending on the airline and the class flown – but if your bag doesn't look too heavy it will rarely be checked.

I do find it rather bizarre that hold baggage weight is checked so carefully, but passengers themselves are not weighed. Airlines would love to do this, even if they didn't charge extra for a particularly heavy passenger or give you a discount for being skinny (though it's a fascinating idea), because having a good idea of the weight on board is important if you want to propel an aircraft safely into the sky.

Without known passenger weights, the airline has to use averages. These vary depending on the point of origin – passengers out of Tokyo, for example, tend to weigh less than those out of Miami. Occasionally this averaging approach causes problems. In the late 1970s a plane was taking off from a German city, headed for London. At the point of rotation, when the plane should leave the ground, it seemed particularly reluctant to take off. The captain tried several times. The end of the runway was looming close – he would have to abandon take-off in seconds. Just in time, the plane bounced off the runway and lumbered painfully slowly into the air.

A disaster had been averted, but it had been close. The plane hadn't seemed to want to take off. After it had landed, heavily but safely, at Heathrow, the plane was checked from end to end. No faults could be found. It was only then that it was discovered that there had been a coin fair on in the city from which the plane took off. Many of the passengers were dealers, carrying their precious coins about their persons. The usual average weights were way too low, and the plane's take-off was put at risk. Maybe weighing passengers

---

Quick Tip: Labelled for Travel

If you want to maximize your chance of keeping your baggage, make sure it is well labelled. Put name, address and contact numbers both inside and outside the bag (inside as well in case the outside tag is lost). If the address is your home one, you may want to make sure that the outside tag is covered – or substitute your office address – so that opportunist thieves can't spot that you are away. Label any bags you intend to carry on the aircraft as well, in case you misplace them or they have to travel in the hold.

wouldn't be such a bad idea after all. For the moment, though, you only have your bags to worry about.

If you need to put some of your bags in the hold, take the precautions used by airline staff. Don't use shiny new suitcases. Instead, disfigure them. Use tape or paint to put large, clear markings on your bags. That way, someone who has exactly the same bag isn't going to grab yours off the carousel before you even get to it – and even if this does happen (occasionally passengers will think the markings were added by baggage handlers) you can spot your luggage being purloined from across a baggage hall.

Don't forget to keep an eye on the weight and size of your hold baggage too. Excess baggage can be expensive, and all too often travellers seem to be surprised when they are charged. Although the check-in agent has a small amount of leeway, and will normally allow you to share out excess baggage weight between a party of travellers, you can expect to be hit if you exceed the limits.

Excess baggage limits vary from airline to airline, so check in advance. As a guideline, these limits are not uncommon: 20 to 23 kg in economy, 30 kg in business class, 40 kg in first class. There are often rather different arrangements for flights to the USA, where there is a tradition of larger allowances. Here you may get away with two bags of up to 32 kg each, provided their total dimensions (length plus height plus width) don't exceed 158 cm. Domestic flights may be restricted to a single bag of this size and weight.

Charges vary hugely. At the time of writing, BA charges fixed rates for the excess items for some routes – for example, £5 for domestic flights and £50 for London to New York – and weight-based rates for others, such as £3.54 per kilogram for London to Rome and £16 per kilogram to get from the UK to Australia. Most airlines will recommend that particularly large or heavy items be sent separately as cargo. If your bags weigh over 40 kg or exceed dimensions of 75 cm by 45 by 95 you will be encouraged to visit the cargo desk.

It is much better if you know in advance that your baggage will have to travel as cargo, as it may take a day or two to catch you up. Phone a number of airline cargo agencies, just as you would shop around for a ticket for yourself. If you don't discover until the day you are flying, it is probably best to stick to the recommendation of the airline you are flying with. Take the baggage along to the cargo desk in the terminal. You should be able to have the bags delivered to your final destination, rather than have to pick them up at the airport, but you will probably find that they take a while to catch you up.

✔ *Checklist: The Hold/Hand Baggage Divide*

How are you going to divide your luggage between hold and hand baggage? Bear in mind that, if possible, you want to get everything into hand baggage, but failing that, here's a suggested split.

Hand Baggage

- ❑ Essential business papers
- ❑ Fragile items – cameras, spectacles, glassware, perishables etc.
- ❑ Books etc. for journey
- ❑ Medication
- ❑ One complete set of clothing
- ❑ Toiletries
- ❑ Travel documents – passport, tickets etc.
- ❑ Valuable items – cash, jewellery, keys etc.

Hold Baggage

- ❑ Papers/books not for journey
- ❑ Bulky items (see maximum hand-baggage size on page 43)
- ❑ Clothes beyond 'first day'
- ❑ Most shoes
- ❑ Nightwear
- ❑ Other items
- ❑ Sharp objects including nail scissors, razor blades, corkscrews and needles

Lock up your essentials

A special form of baggage to consider is a money belt or pouch. Unless you keep your cash, cards and essential documents safe, your trip is liable to turn into a nightmare. A money belt comes into its own on the plane – you may want to hang up your jacket or stow away your handbag, and you are certainly likely to need the toilet at some point. If your essential documents are strapped to your person you needn't worry about them going missing. Ideally you should carry both identification and cash in two locations (this is easier to manage if there are two of you), so that if one set goes missing you will have something to fall back on.

On the plane your main concern will be keeping your documents with you; elsewhere, though, you might want to hide them away entirely. Flashing large amounts of money around in a poor country or district can be asking to be mugged or worse. The less obvious the location of your cash the better. The most popular security devices are money belts or neck pouches which hide the valuables away under the clothing. They are a pain to get at when you need them, but at least they keep things well out of the way. Watch out for discomfort from belts that rub if there's nothing between you and the fabric.

Many holiday travellers resort to bumbags (known as fanny packs in the USA). These have the advantage over a handbag that they are strapped in place, but they are all too easy to open or slash free, so shouldn't be regarded as a security device unless you have the specialist type with a metal-reinforced belt and a complex clasp. In a particularly risky area you might like to carry a decoy wallet with a small amount of cash in it, to produce if you are robbed

Dressing for it

What you wear needs as much thought as your baggage. Physiologically it is a bad move to wear tight clothing on a flight. The low pressure and relative inactivity will make it easy for swelling to cause increased discomfort. This is no time to pretend you can still wear the same collar size as twenty years ago. From a safety viewpoint, it is best not to travel in short skirts, short-sleeved shirts or shorts, which won't give you the protection you need if there is an accident, and to avoid clothes made of particularly flammable substances. Women should bear in mind that this includes tights and stockings, which not only are capable of burning, but also encourage friction burns when sliding down emergency chutes.

There is also a more subtle consideration to bear in mind when considering how to dress. You are, after all, hoping to make the most of your flight. Occasionally there may be the chance of an upgrade. If you are travelling economy, you could be pushed up into business class, or even first. However, the check-in staff usually have an old-fashioned view of what is acceptable for an upgrade. Although your jogging bottoms might be particularly suitable for comfortable travel, you are more likely to get an upgrade if you are wearing a suit or equivalent. You can always change once you've got your seat allocated.

Foot note

When thinking about your clothes, don't forget the vexed question of whether or not to remove your shoes. It is certainly true that feet swell while on board – but this could be seen as a reason for keeping shoes on, or you'll never get them back on at the other end of the flight.

A rule of thumb seems to be to leave them on but to loosen them on a short flight. On a longer flight, take them off and give your feet a chance, but have a pair of shoes that isn't a squeeze to get on, so that at the end of the flight you aren't faced with walking off the aircraft in stockinged feet. Take some slipper socks to keep your own socks protected as you pad around the aisles – spillages are not unusual on aircraft, making the flooring hazardous. Usually in long-haul business and first-class seats you will be given slipper socks as a matter of course.

One way to be ready for landing is to have a pair of travelling shoes that are slightly larger than your normal size. Board the aircraft wearing the shoes with a pair of insoles, so that they come close to fitting. Then take out the insoles before putting your shoes back on at landing.

✔ *Checklist: Comfort Options*

You will face discomfort from tight clothes if you don't take action. Choose the combination of the following that suits you best:

❏ Loosen laces.
❏ Wear oversize shoes with insoles.
❏ Wear loose, slip-on shoes.
❏ Wear espadrilles and other shoes made from floppy materials.
❏ Wear cotton socks (rather than polyester).
❏ Take slippers or slipper socks to wear on board.
❏ Unbutton your collar and waistband.
❏ Wear a shirt with a larger collar size than usual.
❏ Wear trousers with an elasticated waist or button extenders.

Revolution and revolt

One last-minute check is always worth making if you are travelling to any part of the world that isn't 100 per cent safe: ensure that the local political conditions aren't risky. The UK Foreign Office has an excellent web site (see page 327) which includes information from its Travel Advice Unit warning of danger areas which you are recommended not to visit. It's essential reading before you commit yourself to travel. See the same page for the web address of the US State Department, which provides similar information.

First find your terminal

A final element of preparation to consider involves getting to the airport. Make sure that you receive your entitlements. I recently travelled business class to the Far East (someone else was paying), and no one bothered to tell me that I was entitled to a free limousine to the airport. It also pays to make sure that you get to the right place.

One of the delights of my time working at and around London's Heathrow Airport was watching puzzled passengers trying to work out which terminal to aim for and how to get there. Many large airports have several terminals, but Heathrow's arrangements are particularly confusing, as there is no direct access from the three central terminals to Terminal Four and (soon) Terminal Five. It can be quite a shock to discover that you need to take a bus or train ride if you turn up at the wrong terminal.

It is even possible to turn up at the wrong airport if you mistakenly assume that a large city only has one of them. The transit times between sites can easily be over an hour, putting your check-in at risk. If in doubt, consult the airline – and allow even longer than you are told.

✈ *Summary:* **Be Prepared**

- Use a pre-flight checklist (see page 31).

- Check immunization requirements in plenty of time.

- Ensure that you are medically fit to fly.

- Don't forget visa requirements.

- Plan your cash needs.

- Check the conditions at your destination.

- Travel light – use only hand baggage if possible.

- Make your suitcases easy to recognize.

- Dress for comfort.

3 At the Airport

So, you have arrived at the airport. For some, the nightmare is just about to begin. A well-known travel writer likens airports to shopping malls from hell. Whereas the shopping mall is (supposedly) designed to make you feel comfortable and relaxed, encouraging you to stay longer and spend more, airports seem purpose-built to maximize stress and unpleasantness.

De-stressing the airport

As someone who for many years worked at one of the world's worst airports for generating stress (London Heathrow), I can assure you that there is, in fact, no malice involved. Occasionally there is a degree of inconvenience designed in, though. When Heathrow's Terminal Four was built it was decided that friends and family spent too long at the airport seeing off their loved ones. These non-travellers were clogging up limited short-term parking and generally getting in the way. Because of this, Terminal Four was designed with very little of interest in the check-in hall compared with the other Heathrow terminals – all the rest is behind the passengers-only gate. This apart, the unfriendliness of airports is largely due to accident rather than design.

It doesn't help that the mild undercurrent of fear makes flying inherently stressful. But the airport and the airlines are also obliged to go through a range of processes to get your bags to the right place, to keep out terrorists, and to comply with the bewildering range of regulations that must be followed. Most of the discomfort and chaos of airport life has evolved naturally rather than being planned.

Even so, the whole atmosphere – people in a hurry, crowds, queues, harsh fluorescent lighting, vast echoing halls making the already high level of noise even more irritating – conspires to make the airport experience an unpleasant one. Perhaps the best advice on how to cope with the stress of the airport is not to make it worse by adding your own stress to the picture.

The simplest way to minimize stress is to arrive with plenty of time. Experienced travellers may raise an eyebrow at the sheep who really believe the airline when it says you need to check in three hours before the flight (or whatever), but the fact is that this buffer time is just as valuable for you as it is for the carrier. It means you aren't going to be fazed by a traffic jam on the airport motorway, a sudden absence of trains on the express rail link, or just getting out of bed a bit late. There is certainly nothing to make the whole stress of the airport environment worse than turning up late and having to find your way around a confusing maze of a building with minutes to spare.

I recently saw a businessman turn up at London's Luton Airport. He arrived too late to check in, though the flight had not yet taken off. He was furious with the airline, but all its staff could do was point out that it was his responsibility to get to the airport on time – there was nothing the airline could do about his delays. In his case it had taken three hours to travel the 56 km from central London to Luton. However long you think it will take, allow a little more.

Quick Tip: **Telephone Check-in**

If you are stuck in a traffic jam and the minutes are ticking away towards your flight departure, use a mobile phone to telephone the airline. Explain your circumstances, and see if it can check you in over the phone. If you have only hand baggage, this will mean that you can head straight for the gate and cut precious minutes off your timing when you arrive. Remember also to ask for directions for getting from the drop-off point to the gate.

This tip is usable only if you have a mobile phone and the number of the airline with you – don't leave home without either.

Getting to the airport on time can sometimes be harder when you are in a strange place and dependent on others for your timings. For safety, you might like to add a half hour or so to any timings you are given by local experts, or to catch the bus or train before the one that was recommended. It's much better to be just a bit too early than be faced with the possibility of being stranded in a strange location. The ideal seems to be to get yourself through all the busy processes as quickly as possible, then find yourself a haven of calm – the departure lounge, the executive lounge (more on that in a moment), the shops – anywhere that you personally find de-stressing.

It all went wrong

The point at which you arrive at the airport is the most likely time to discover that you have made a mistake. Talk to any airline customer-contact staff and you will discover a whole list of ways in which passengers manage to mess things up, but the most frequent problems tend to be forgetting documentation and excessive baggage weights. If you have taken the sensible precautions of the previous chapter there shouldn't be any problems, but we all slip up occasionally.

Now is not the time to get angry with the airline repre-sentative – you are going to need all the help you can get. Most of the regulations are there for very good reasons of security or the practicalities of flying an aircraft. The every-day nature of flight tends to conceal the fact that it isn't as simple as a bus journey. To achieve a safe trip through what is a very hostile environment, the airline has to be very fussy about all the little details.

First and foremost of the troublesome documents is the lost or forgotten passport. You can expect plenty of sympathy from the customer-service agent, and if you take a constructive approach rather than shouting you may be given free use of a phone to try to get a friend or relation to bring the passport over to the airport, but don't expect any leeway on this one. Not only does the airline have a legal obligation to make sure that you have the right documents to travel, it will be subject to a large fine if it gets it wrong.

Expect to have your passport given attention both at check-in and at the gate. If you haven't got it, there really is no point making a fuss – you cannot make an international trip, full stop. If you have lost your passport while abroad, you will need to get special documentation from your embassy or consulate. Realistically, you are not going to get your flight, so you might as well accept it.

The same applies to the rather more murky area of visas. As much as possible, the airline will also check that you meet any visa requirements (again, it is liable to be fined for any mistakes). Very occasionally, under special circumstances, visa requirements can be slightly modified. This can happen only if the airline can get a fax with permission from the immigration department of the country concerned. You can expect this only if you have a truly impressive reason (it has been done, for example, for Olympic athletes who didn't have appropriate visas). On the whole, though, a missing visa is nearly as bad as a missing passport.

Ticketless travel

The other document you could mislay or have stolen is your ticket. Here things aren't quite as bad, though you will need to allow plenty of time at the airport to get things sorted out. (If you find out in advance, ring the company's office and make arrangements beforehand.) In principle, as the e-ticket demonstrates, there is no reason why a ticket should be needed. The definitive record of your booking is not the piece of paper but the entry in the airline's reservation system. All you should need is a means of proving that you are the person for whom the reservation was made. For at least twenty years airlines have been talking about widespread ticketless flight; however, it remains the exception rather than the rule.

As soon as you discover that you have lost your ticket, inform the airline and the police (if there's a possibility that the ticket was stolen). It helps a lot to have details of your booking reference – the sequence of characters that identifies your reservation. Even without this, the agent should be able to find your details, but keeping the reference jotted down somewhere will make things a lot easier for everyone. Before replacing your ticket, the airline has the right to charge you an administration charge – this could be anything from around £10 to £100.

The reason why lost tickets are such a problem is that the ticket itself constitutes a negotiable document, a bit like a cheque or a money order. This means it isn't possible for the airline simply to replace the piece of paper, any more than you would expect a bank to replace a £10 note that you dropped in the street. The airline will issue you with a new ticket, but has every right to charge you for that ticket at whatever the going rate is at that time. (Bear in mind that airline tickets get more expensive as you get closer to the date of flight, so it may well be more than you paid.) The agent may waive this charge if it will cause you difficulties, provided you sign an indemnity agreeing to pay for the second ticket if the lost one is subsequently cashed in.

If you do have to pay for the second ticket, the good news is that, assuming both tickets don't get used, you will normally be able to get a refund, and the refund should be for the cost of the more expensive ticket. The bad news is that it can take a long time for the refund to come through. Full-price airline tickets can be cashed in after the flight for up to a year, so the airline may wait until the unused ticket has expired before giving you your money back. A few airlines simply won't refund a lost ticket at all (US carrier Southwest Airlines is one). They are perfectly within their rights – the whole legal basis of air carriage is biased heavily in favour of the airlines.

It went without me

If the worst comes to the worst and you miss your flight, for whatever reason, your first priority is to see what the alternatives are.

→ Fast Track:
Left Behind

Some essentials to consider when you have missed a flight:

- When is the next flight?

- Can I use another airline's flights?

- Can I get a flight from another airport quicker?

- For a short flight, can I use alternatives (train, taxi, bus) rather than flying?

- What am I going to do between now and the new departure time?

- Will I have to pay to transfer to another flight?

- Is it worth travelling at all now?

Before spending a lot of effort on getting to your destination, make sure that you really need to do so. If not catching the flight makes you miss out on the main reason for travelling, you might do better to contact the people at the other end and reschedule the whole thing (if this is possible) rather than go through the often painful process of getting a later flight.

Assuming you do need to travel, make sure you examine all the possible ways of getting to your destination – don't assume that you will simply rebook on the same airline's next available flight. Go to the airline's information desk and get it to check your options. If it was your fault that you missed the flight, throw yourself on the airline's mercy – make it clear you know it was your fault, but explain the difficult circumstances. You may find at the very least that it waives any rebooking fee.

If missing the flight was anyone other than the airline's fault, there is no point trying to blame the airline. It is not going to take responsibility for the fact that your bus broke down. Again, play for sympathy, but don't get angry. If the fault belongs to the airline itself you can be firmer and more assertive. As we will see, airlines have few obligations even when the fault is theirs, but they are more likely to be flexible if they can be shown to be at fault.

Even if the problem is your fault, you may find that the airline is prepared to be helpful. Ask what it can do. If you need to stay in a hotel at your own expense to catch the next flight, ask the airline to make the booking – it should be able to get a discount for you as a 'distressed passenger'.

→ Fast Track:
Not Getting Left Behind

It's better to plan ahead and avoid missing a flight. Take these precautions:

- Bear in mind that airlines don't guarantee their schedules. Allow for delays in connections when you plan your trip.

- Watch out for connections involving airports where bad weather (snow, fog etc.) are likely to cause delays – if necessary, look for a different route.

- When making a connection between the flights of two different airlines, ask both airlines to make a note of your connecting details in their PNR (Passenger Name Record) – the computer record that contains your details. If you are delayed, they may be able to take steps to get you through the airport as quickly as possible.

- If you are delayed and miss your flight, don't stand in a long queue to rebook – use a phone and call the airline's reservation number to jump the queue.

- If you are flying on an e-ticket and need to change airlines, ask the original carrier to print out a conventional ticket or endorse your ticket before going to the new one.

- If your flight is late and a following connection is at risk, tell the agent at the gate if you are yet to board. If you are already on the plane, let a member of the cabin crew know. They will contact the airport to warn them of your late arrival, or at the very least, get you off the plane first.

- If you need to make a connection quickly at an unfamiliar airport, check the in-flight magazine for maps and ask cabin crew for guidance – you might save precious minutes.

The check-in challenge

There's an element of 'us versus them' when you reach the check-in desk. It's a competition between you and the staff. You want to avoid queues, get checked in quickly, select your ideal seat, and be given an upgrade. The staff want a

hassle-free process, ideally without talking to any customers. (Actually, that isn't fair. Many check-in agents
enjoy talking to the right kind of passengers – that's to say,
passengers that don't cause any trouble.)

The first challenge comes when you approach the desk.
Often there will be several desks checking in the same
flight. If you have an economy ticket, should you join the
end of the huge queue – every person seemingly carrying at
least ten pieces of luggage and prepared to argue indefinitely over excess-baggage costs – or do you slip in at the
business-class check-in, where there is only one other
passenger?

The first observation is that it is perfectly possible to get
away with doing the latter. Most check-in agents will check
in economy passengers at a business-class desk if there is a
queue for economy and none for them. They don't particularly like messy queues in front of the desk, and are happy
to help out their colleagues to clear away the passengers.
But – and it's a big but – the action is at the check-in
agent's discretion.

Learn from my experience a number of years ago. I was
consulting on the usability of a new computer system to
help with check-in. As part of the process of becoming
more familiar with check-in itself, I was allowed to sit
behind a check-in desk for a morning and play at being a
check-in agent, while the real thing looked over my
shoulder. I had been told that it was OK to check in
economy passengers if we had a lull, and mid-morning I
did just that, only to be told off in no uncertain terms by
my mentor agent.

What no one had mentioned to me was that I had to apply a few quick visual criteria to the people wanting to check in. They had to look respectable, not like students or backpackers. I had committed the sin of checking in a long-haired man with a rucksack at business class. There were two reasons given for this policy. One was to make sure that the business-class check-in area looked smart in case a real business-class traveller turned up. The other was that word got round 'that kind of person' faster, so we were likely to end up with every backpacker jumping out of the queues and flocking to the business-class desk.

You may or may not agree with the policy, based as it is on stereotypes, but this is the approach that is likely to be taken. If you want to slip around the queues, make

---

Quick Tip: Departure Tax

Many countries charge an airport departure tax. This is collected at check-in, and often has to be paid in local currency. Make sure that you have enough cash with you at the end of a trip to deal with this. The Worldwise web site (see page 327) has information on the levels of departure tax in different countries.

If you are travelling business or first class, the airline will often pay the departure tax for you. Check beforehand, so you aren't landed with an unnecessary handful of local currency. You won't be able to do a lot with, say, 40 Malaysian ringgits if you end up taking them home.

yourself look conventionally respectable – no brightly dyed hair, bare feet, obvious body-piercing beyond conventional earrings for women, no T-shirts and jeans, and no ruck-sacks and carrier bags (other than designer labels). That way you have a great chance of legitimately jumping the queue. Don't, of course, demand this as a right. Ask in a slightly pathetic way, 'Can I check in here for *wherever*?' Make it clear that you know that the person in uniform is the boss, and throw yourself on his or her mercy.

Bye-bye bags

As you check in, if you have taken my advice, you won't have any hold baggage to say goodbye to – but realistically it is not practicable always to rely on hand luggage. If you have to send bags off to the hold, there are a couple of essentials to make sure that your bags are properly treated.

A first, simple check is that the bags are going to the right destination. Check that the baggage tags have the correct code (see Appendix 8 – page 341). Second, hang on to your stubs. For each bag you should be given a small label that will be attached to your ticket. Make sure you keep this safe. If for any reason a bag goes missing, this is your proof that the bag existed. Don't discard the label with your used travel documents until the bag is safely in your hands and you have checked that the contents are as you left them.

The overbooking syndrome

Imagine this. You arrive at the airport with a firm ticket for a scheduled airline and with plenty of time. After a few minutes' strolling around the airport shops you cross over to check-in. The small queue seems to be moving very slowly. Everyone is arguing with the check-in agent. By the time you reach the front of the queue you have already overheard what is wrong, but you can't really believe it, so you have to hear it again for yourself. The flight is over-booked. The airline has sold more seats than are available on the plane, and some passengers are not going to leave on this flight – it's simple arithmetic.

Before looking at your rights, we need to find out why a (presumably) respectable business like your airline would have sold seats it hadn't got? The answer lies in the nature of the ticket. While many low-cost tickets are subject to a host of restrictions, full-fare tickets have a near-unique quality. They are refundable after the event if you don't use them. It's bizarre really. No one would expect to be able to refund a ticket to a show after the event if they didn't get round to attending it. But, as we have already seen, full-fare airline tickets are almost the equivalent of a money order.

Because of this feature of the product, buyers with plenty of cash to spare – companies, for example – can get round the inconvenience of booking for a particular flight. If, for instance, an executive wants to fly from New York to London tomorrow, but doesn't know when, the company can buy half a dozen tickets, use the one that matches the arrival time at the airport, and get a refund on the rest. Weighing time against money, the convenience can be worth the marginal expenditure for the time that the tickets are held.

But this gives the airlines a headache. On some routes as many as a third, or even a half, of the passengers booked on a flight aren't going to show up. So big airlines spend a small fortune predicting how many passengers won't turn up on a particular route, on a particular date, at a particular time. This prediction is used to set an 'overbooking profile' – for example, if you think you may have fifty passengers not show up, you might sell (say) thirty-five more tickets than the plane can hold. And more than 95 per cent of the time everything will be fine. But in the end such predictions can only ever be a sophisticated guess. Sometimes more passengers than expected will arrive at check-in and the result is overbooking.

Benefiting from overbooking

So the airline tells you that there aren't enough seats to go round. It will usually start proceedings by trying to buy off some of the passengers with cash or travel vouchers in return for waiting for a later flight. If you aren't in any hurry, this isn't a bad position to be in. The airline will offer you a reward for the inconvenience of being removed from your flight (known as being bumped in the trade).

Before accepting the airline's offer, get a clear picture of how you are going to end up. Check when the next flight is, and whether or not you will get a confirmed seat on it. Check just what the airline is willing to offer in the way of comfort. If you are bumped and need to wait a fair amount of time, it is worth trying to get a catering voucher out of the staff member. (These vouchers are discretionary, so it pays to be nice, rather than 'Mr/Ms Angry'.) If it's evening time, what about a hotel room? And bear in mind that there is no official minimum or maximum to the financial incentive that can be offered. Be prepared to haggle – but bear in mind that the staff making the transaction probably have limits imposed by the airline. If part of the offer is a free ticket or voucher, check any restrictions that may apply to it to see just how valuable it is to you.

Perhaps in your particular case you have to travel now. Yet the airline has failed to squeeze out enough excess passengers. It decides that, as you were among the last to check in and not an exalted member of its frequent-flier club, you will be excluded from the flight. What are your options? First, get in the right frame of mind. You may be furious with the airline for what it has done to you, but the person on the check-in desk or at the gate is *not* personally responsible. He or she did not see you coming and decide to dump the problem on you. So don't take it out on the only person who may be able to help.

There's an even better reason for being as pleasant as you can. The airline has very few obligations to you. Thanks to the Warsaw Convention (see page 249), having an airline ticket gives you very few rights. Any advantage you can gain will be at the discretion of the agent you are about to deal with. So think motivational. Try to make your position 'us versus them' – get the agent to side with you. Be sympathetic (but don't waste time – there might be a big queue). Explain why you have to get to your destination so soon, and ask if there are any seats in the next class up that you might be able to use. It's not that you are angling for an upgrade (though that would be a nice plus), just that you need to fly.

If the desk is set up so you can see its computer screen, you may even be able to check this for yourself. There will usually be a seating display that lists the number of seats booked and checked in for the various classes. Look for a positive availability in first class (usually F or P) or business (look for C or J). If you do spot some seats, don't lose your advantage by storming in and demanding one, but you can keep up your positive, assertive requests with more confidence.

If no matter what you do you can't make any headway and are still prevented from flying, there are a number of options open to you. Check our complaints chapter on page 245.

For US airlines only, there are strict rules on what happens if they overbook a flight and they can't get enough volunteers to wait for a later flight. The US Department of Transport specifies the following requirements for passengers who are bumped from a flight against their will:

- If the airline can come up with an alternative that will get you to your destination (including onward connections) within one hour of your scheduled time, there is no compensation.

- With between one and two hours' delay, the airline must pay you the equivalent of a one-way fare to your final destination, up to a maximum of $200.

- Over two hours' delay (four hours for international flights) and the compensation is twice a one-way fare, up to a maximum of $400.

Note that this is compensation for your inconvenience. You still get to keep your original ticket, either to use later or to get a refund – the airline is obliged to pay up. This compensation doesn't apply if the airline is bumping you because it had to substitute a smaller plane, if your ticket isn't confirmed, if you pay late, or if you check in late. It doesn't apply to charter flights, aircraft seating fewer than sixty passengers, and international flights other than those leaving from the USA. But at least it's something.

Within the European Union there is now some degree of protection as well. The exact amount varies from airline to airline, but, as a guideline, British Airways offers £150 for a short-haul flight and £200 for a long-haul flight – though this is in vouchers rather than as cash. Watch out for limitations on these vouchers. Elsewhere it is down to the local country's rules. Tread carefully when demanding your rights.

Before making involuntary bumps, the airline will usually look for volunteers. Officially the policy is usually to give exactly the same compensation to volunteers, but you may find that you can haggle an improvement, as the staff would rather that they did not have to irritate passengers by bumping them against their will.

→ Fast Track:
  Dealing with the Desk

All too often, passengers who face uniformed staff on the other side of a desk resort to anger if problems arise. A shouting match will not get you the best results. Here are five simple things that work better:

• Instead of shouting, speak calmly. Take a few deep breaths first if you feel you aren't going to manage this.

• Instead of showing your distaste, smile. Everyone responds better to a smile.

• Instead of getting angry, get assertive. Don't give in – keep restating your case, but always calmly and pleasantly.

• Instead of relating history, stick to the point. It is tempting to tell the person behind your desk all your woes, but by keeping to the point you want something done about you are more likely to achieve a good result.

• Instead of commanding, ask. Although good customer-service staff will not show too much resentment at being told what to do, they will all respond better to a polite request rather than a blunt demand.

Choosing the seat

Either when you make your booking or at check-in you are going to have to choose a seat. Generally the airline will allocate one. The computer selects a seat that is most appropriately positioned to balance the load on the aircraft. This isn't necessary for safety, but if there's no other reason for selecting a seat the plane may as well be evenly balanced.

Don't feel that you have to take the seat that has been allocated. It is no problem for the check-in agent to make a change. In choosing a seat, you have several decisions to make, though you may be offered only one or two choices up front – it is up to you to take the initiative on anything else. If smoking is allowed on the flight, you will be asked if you want a smoking or a non-smoking seat. If at all possible, *even if you are a smoker*, I would recommend avoiding smoking flights. See page 105 for more details, but smoking on board both increases the risk of fire and significantly reduces the oxygen content in what is already thin air. Vote with your feet on the matter of smoking flights.

If you have no choice, bear in mind that smoke is no respecter of arbitrary divisions. By the end of a long smoking flight, despite air filters and the rest, there will be a visible fug throughout the cabin. You can certainly request a seat as far away as possible from smoking, but don't expect miracles.

The other choice that you will usually be offered is an aisle or a window seat (very few people actually choose to sit in one of the seats in between, unless they are travelling in a party). Having this choice is one of the reasons for checking in a reasonable time ahead of departure – late arrivals are likely to be left with those undesirable 'piggy in the middle' seats. Generally speaking I would recommend the aisle seat, particularly on a long journey where to get out into the aisle you would have to climb over another passenger who was trying to sleep. If you intend to stretch your legs regularly – a valuable aid to avoiding deep-vein thrombosis (see page 93) – being in the aisle seat has obvious advantages.

In principle, in a confined economy-class seat, the aisle position also gives you a chance to stretch out your legs, though it is essential to be wary of the trolleys that will be trundled up and down the aisles with only centimetres of clearance to spare. The only real disadvantage to being in the aisle seat is that you suffer from your fellow passengers trying to get past, and you are directly underneath the overhead lockers, and so need to keep a wary eye open when they are unlatched, just in case a piece of luggage has been shifted around by the aircraft's climb or turbulence and is waiting to plummet down on to you.

A different choice that the check-in agent probably won't put to you is between one of the side rows or the centre block. On a wide-bodied jet there can be as many as five seats together in the centre of the aircraft. Although there will never be more than two people between you and the aisle, this feels much more hemmed in than the seating in the side rows and should be avoided unless you are travelling with a number of companions and want to be seated together. As seats are lettered from the left-hand side (facing the front of the aircraft), on a wide-bodied jet the left section will generally be seats A to C, the centre D to H, and the right-hand side J to L (there isn't an I, to avoid confusion with the number one). If you have any doubts about where the seat you are offered is, ask. The check-in agent won't mind.

Another interesting challenge is to decide on which seats to choose if two of you are travelling together. It might seem sensible on an outside row of three seats to take (say) the aisle and the middle seat, so that you will be seated together. However, a much better tactic is to take the window and aisle seats. That way you minimize the possibility of having to share your space with someone else. If you do end up with someone in between, ask them to swap – they would nearly always prefer a window or aisle seat, and there is no obligation to stay in the seat that you have been allocated. When I first started flying, many years ago, I endured a flight from London to Chicago sandwiched between two wartime GI brides who had been on a nostalgic trip back to their home town of Newcastle upon Tyne. They were lovely ladies, and their meld of Newcastle and Chicago accents was fascinating, but we would all have been more comfortable if we had realized we could have swapped.

If your flight is on the long-haul workhorse the Boeing 747, you may have one other decision to make – whether to go for the upper deck or the lower. Usually this option is available to business-class passengers, though some airlines use upstairs for extra economy seating. Putting safety aside for a moment, the upper deck can be more pleasant. It is less confining than the space below, and, as in the first-class cabin, there is a feeling of spaciousness because there is nothing in front of you (except the flight deck). It also seems in the business-class layout that the two toilets upstairs tend to be less heavily utilized than the ones down below. Because of the layout, it also feels as if you are getting more attention from the staff too.

There is not enough evidence to determine whether travelling upstairs is less safe than the lower deck. It feels subjectively more risky, because there are only two emergency exits available as against the four that serve the business-class cabin below, and because you are higher off the ground, but I have not been able to find any definitive statistics to determine the safety factor either way.

The final decision is whether or not to go for a special row. Not all seats on the aircraft are identical. Sometimes there will be a row that doesn't recline, perhaps backing on to a bulkhead, one of the dividing walls between the sections of the aircraft. These seats are best avoided – you can always ask the check-in agent to make sure you haven't got one of them. On the positive side, there will be two types of row where you can win yourself more space. The first comprises the seats that face on to a bulkhead. Here you will have a little more legroom, and, crucially, you will not have a seat in front of you that gets reclined into your face – your space remains your own in a bulkhead seat.

There is a price for this luxury, though. Because there is no seat in front, there is nothing to put your cabin bag under, so you are restricted on the size of bag you can stow away. This problem is particularly acute on the upper deck of 747s, where the overhead lockers are usually smaller than on the lower deck. If your hand baggage won't fit in the locker, the crew will tuck it away somewhere for you, but this is less convenient during the flight.

There is one circumstance where you may prefer the window seat, despite the inconvenience of scrambling over the person next to you. Under the windows of the upper deck there are often storage bins which take more than the overhead lockers. Also, the crew may overlook a bag on the floor by your feet in a bulkhead seat if it is tucked away against the wall of the aircraft – something that is possible only in the window seat.

The other type of special row is situated next to an emergency exit. Here there has to be extra space between your seat and the one in front, so even in the economy cabin there's a fair amount of space to stretch your legs. You also have the advantage that in the unlikely event of an emergency you are not going to have to fight your way through a smoky cabin to get to the exit. Perhaps less encouraging is the fact you will have to be extra careful about not strewing your bits and pieces on the floor, sometimes seats in this row do not recline, and you will need to be capable of opening the emergency exit and of helping people off the plane if anything goes wrong. For this reason there are a number of passengers who simply can't sit there. If you have a baby, if you have trouble lifting (emergency exits weigh around 25 kg), if you are in a wheelchair or if you don't speak the appropriate language well enough then the emergency-exit row is not for you.

Whichever seat you choose, with check-in completed you will normally have time on your hands. But rather than hang around in the airport departures hall, however tempting it is if you are being seen off by friends and relations, it makes sense to get through the remaining hurdles that the airport puts in your way before relaxing.

→ Fast Track:
Getting the Best Seat

• Frequent fliers will often get a better choice of seat on crowded flights.

• Try to get your preferred seat allocated at the time you make your booking.

• The later you leave your seat selection, the less likely you are to get the best seats. Aisle seats go first, followed by window seats.

• Exit-row seats can't be reserved – the check-in staff need to see you. If you want one of these, get to check-in early and ask for it.

• If the seats you want are hard to come by, try calling the airline's reservations just after midnight. Any unpaid reservations will just have been cancelled, so new seats might become available.

• You don't have to stay in your allocated seat once on board. As soon as the seat-belt sign goes off you can move (though the cabin crew would prefer it if you ask first).

• Sitting behind the engines tends to be rather noisier, and the back of the plane is most sensitive to turbulence.

- If travelling with someone with a better frequent-flier/executive-club status, get them to make the booking. If you want to sit together, ask for a window/aisle pair of seats, and the centre seat will only be allocated as a last resort.

- Alternatively, ask for two adjacent aisle seats.

Gate games

Check-in is usually the point where you find out which gate you are to fly from, though you may have to wait until the gate is allocated if you arrive particularly early. In later parts of the book we will explore the statistics of flight safety, but it is worth stating at this point that there is no linkage between a particular gate number and risk for the flight – so there really is no point in going out of your way to avoid gate 13.

Many airports don't have a gate 13, to prevent customers from worrying, but this can result in concerns about gate 14, on the assumption that somehow this is 'really' gate 13. There is no need for concern – the statistics bear out that gate number is irrelevant to flight safety. Interestingly, Heathrow's Terminal Four was specifically designed with gates 12 and 14 at opposite ends of the building, to make it less obvious that gate 13 does not exist.

Making it through security

Check-in is not your last challenge before making it to the plane. There is still security to come. No one with any common sense is going to deny the value of airport security. The appalling consequences of getting it wrong have been made clear in the past. The delays introduced by security are a necessary price to pay to reduce the risks from terrorism. However, this doesn't mean you have to enjoy the process – security is rarely fun, and always demands a trade-off between protection and convenience.

This lack of fun goes with the territory. Don't be tempted to lighten the moment and inject a touch of comedy into this miserable process. Even though security guards have as good a sense of humour as anyone else, they are not prepared to extend it into their work. There is a useful lesson in the experience of the Canadian violinist flying from London Heathrow who featured in the BBC's popular *Airport* fly-on-the-wall documentary series. When asked about his violin case, this unfortunate traveller found the question, 'What is in it?' so crass that he thought he would lighten the moment by saying, 'A machine gun.' All he intended was a light-hearted reference to the way that 1920s Chicago mobsters used violin cases as convenient disguises for their weapons. Unfortunately, the security guard was in no mood for a joke, and the bewildered violinist was arrested and taken to the airport police station. Although he was not eventually charged, he missed his flight and had a very unpleasant experience for anyone in a foreign country.

It simply isn't worth the risk of trying to be funny. Don't make references to weapons, bombs, terrorists or hijacks, even in an undertone or a whisper. Think before you speak. There is an apocryphal story that a traveller was once arrested for calling out to a friend he had just spotted across the departure lounge. His ill-thought-out cry of 'Hi, Jack!' got him in big trouble.

Being zapped

Security may be an essential, but there is potential for the facilities used to check for concealed weapons to cause damage. Heart pacemakers and similar devices can be affected by the powerful magnetic fields in the metal-detector arches that all passengers are expected to pass through. In theory in many countries (including the UK, the USA and most of Europe) the magnetic fields are specially devised to keep pacemakers safe, but if you have such a device fitted it is always worth explaining the fact and asking for a physical search instead. It is an inconvenience, but nowhere near as bad as the possible outcome if you pass through the arch and it damages your medical device.

If you have metal medical implants (pins, screws, plates etc.) you are not at risk from the device, but you may well trigger it. It is worth carrying a letter from your medical team explaining this – you will probably still be subjected to a hand search, but it will mean that the security staff understand why you have triggered the machine and so may be less suspicious.

As a passenger walks through the arch, his or her hand baggage will be travelling on a conveyor belt through an X-ray machine. Almost always the staff will cheerfully tell you that the X-ray machine won't damage film – but there is good evidence that some machines muddy the pictures on faster films (those with the higher ASA numbers – anything above around 200 for safety). Put your films in a separate bag and ask for it to be hand-checked. I have seen lead-lined bags for sale to protect your film, but these seem pointless, as the security guard is bound to want to know what's in them, so you will still have to go through a manual check.

I am much less convinced of the possibility of damage to laptops and other electronic devices by exposure to X-rays. While most security guards will hand-check PCs, it can be tedious as you will need to switch on the laptop and prove it isn't a dummy. The only obvious risk is that the mechanism required to produce X-rays requires high voltages, and this can mean strong magnetic fields. Hopefully these will be well screened inside the device (in fact, if anything, there may be more danger of magnetic damage by passing a laptop or floppy disks close to the outside of a machine, where there may be less shielding against magnetic influence). If you do want to go for a hand check, it is best to remove the laptop, shove the bag on the X-ray-machine belt, and then present the guard with a naked device. This makes it unlikely that he or she will argue that it should pass through the scanner.

It may seem obvious, but time after time passengers set off the security arch's metal-detector because they haven't emptied their pockets. If possible, put the obvious items like loose coins and your mobile phone in the bag that goes through the scanner – otherwise remember to drop them in the box or basket provided before you head through the arch. Remember to remove metal-framed spectacles as well. It is worth it to avoid a slow hand search.

The scanner scam

Wherever you are in an airport terminal your baggage is at risk. You only have to look around the concourse to see hundreds of well-stuffed bags and briefcases asking to be stolen. Their owners are distracted by the environment, unfamiliar with exactly where they are going, and can easily lose concentration. Do you know, for example, exactly what is happening to your hand baggage while you check in? If it's a shoulder bag, keep it on your shoulder (this also reduces the chance that the check-in agent will question its size and weight). If it isn't, position a foot firmly on a strap or the bag itself.

But for the suspicious traveller (the only sensible kind), being in the vicinity of the X-ray scanner should make you particularly wary of what is happening to your bags. Watch them as they pass into the X-ray machine. Tampering can occur as other people add items to the belt – perhaps they will decide to use your bag to smuggle through a dangerous item. It is also one of the most frequent occasions when bags get stolen. Usually the sensible traveller will have his or her bags to hand at all times. But when you pass through security you will be letting go of your bag and heading off through a separate archway. You are at your most vulnerable.

At this point, clever thieves – often operating in pairs – can strike. They usually work something like this. The two thieves get in front of a likely target in the check-in queue. They particularly like the shoulder bags used to carry a laptop computer – it's a fair bet that there will be an expensive item inside – so, even if like me you find these bags make a useful alternative to a briefcase, they are probably best avoided. The first thief passes quickly through the detector arch. The second thief follows behind. By now your bag is on the conveyor through the scanner. The first thief is through the metal detector. The accomplice passes through – and sets off the alarm.

Everyone's attention is taken by the alarm. You are held up as the accomplice messes about, perhaps deliberately misunderstanding what is going on. And the first thief calmly walks off with your bag. It isn't just the security guards that need to be vigilant. Whatever happens, keep your eye on your bag from putting it on to the X-ray conveyor to picking it up at the other side. Be prepared to yell. Even better, if you are travelling with a companion, do your own working in pairs, keeping an eye on each other's bags.

Lounging about

At most airports each large airline has a lounge for its special passengers – a haven of peace with a more relaxing atmosphere than the general hustle and bustle of the intricate web of passageways, shops, offices and gates that makes up the airside component of an airport. Unlike the doubtful promise of comfort and service on the aircraft, always limited by practicality, most airline lounges really are very pleasant places to be. Assuming you have managed to get the essential airport business out of the way, I have no doubt that these are the best places to spend the time you have to spare before boarding the plane.

The seats are much more comfortable than those in any open lounge, and there will be convenient drinks and snacks – plenty to keep hunger at bay even on a wait of several hours – and a range of ways to keep your attention distracted from the less pleasant aspects of flying. You will be kept informed of the status of your flight, and if you need some last-minute business facilities, like a fax or Internet access, they will usually be available. There are even showers in most lounges, so that you can refresh yourself on a long journey. The question is not whether or not to try to get in a lounge, but why you aren't there already.

Usually those flying on first-class or business-class tickets will have automatic access to a lounge, but these aren't the only way to get in. Some of the airlines' frequent-flier clubs and executive clubs allow even a humble economy passenger to make use of a lounge as a result of membership. The airline's main reason for operating these clubs is to get to know their customers better – it's an exercise in relationship marketing. But, for the members, benefits like lounges far outweigh the small fee that may be involved for membership. If you travel several times a year and don't already belong, it is probably worth adding a few clubs to your armoury.

I would say that, apart from space on the aircraft, access to a lounge is the single biggest reason for paying the extortionate business-class fare. If you aren't travelling business class and don't have appropriate club membership it might be worth throwing yourself on the mercy of the check-in agent who issues the 'invitation' to the lounge. Check-in staff can be rather more forgiving than those at the entrance to the lounge, who tend to take a very sniffy view of anyone without the right credentials. Sell yourself appropriately to an agent on a quiet check-in desk and you may be able to bypass the requirements.

You can't pay the airline to get in the lounge (except by buying a business-class ticket), but in some cities there are now airport-run lounges where any passenger can appreciate the benefits of a lounge for an appropriate fee.

Getting to the plane

When the flight is called, it's fine not to appear inexperienced. There's no need to jump into the air and head for the gate as soon as you hear boarding announced. But, equally, don't leave it too late. Make sure you know how long it takes to get from the lounge to the gate – at some airports you have to allow as much as fifteen or twenty minutes for this. Cut it too fine and the captain will make the decision to offload your bags. Once this happens, you are off the flight whether or not the doors are actually closed. (This is another reason why it's good to have only hand baggage.) It's much better to get on the plane reasonably early, so you can find your seat and get settled in without having to squeeze yourself through hordes of other passengers.

Of course, boarding is often by row, so you may not be able to get on straight away. Here's another advantage of travelling business or first. Once boarding starts, you can get on whenever you like. If you have one of these tickets, make sure you take advantage of the fast-track options available to you. On a recent long-haul trip I saw several fellow business-class travellers join a long queue to enter the gate lounge. They hadn't spotted that the premium passengers had their own desk slightly further along the corridor with no queue at all.

Similarly, once in the gate lounge, there was a long string of passengers waiting, sheeplike, to go down the second air bridge to the back of the aircraft. There was no one using the front air bridge, and no one there to say that business-class passengers should use it. It felt as if I was breaking some rule or other as I took the long walk alone down the bridge, but in fact it was what the crew expected. If you are paying that much, make sure you get the benefits.

Connections

Before entirely finishing with the airport, it is worth spending a moment on that most stressful of departures, the connection. If you need to fly into one airport with the sole intention of flying straight out again, it is very tempting to schedule the arrival and departure as close as possible, to avoid wasting your time. However, you have to bear in mind the realistic delays that may occur. Even the aircraft taking a different taxiway between the runway and the terminal can introduce unexpected minutes into a journey time.

When booking a connecting flight, you should check with the airline just what is involved in making the connection. Bear in mind that at some airports you will need to change terminals – at Heathrow, for example, arriving on a long-haul flight and leaving on a short-haul can mean a good half-hour's journey just to get between terminals. The airline should be able to recommend a connection time at a particular airport, but that's all it will be – a recommendation.

If your on-time arrival is absolutely essential, it makes sense either to look for a non-stop flight or to have a break in the intermediate city, so you can use an overnight stay as a buffer to cope with any problems on the first leg. If you are prepared to take on the risk of connections, you can expect much more sympathy from an airline if you are making a connection at the airline's own recommended timing than if you have made your own tight schedule. By keeping to the airline's recommendations you should be able to be moved to an alternative flight at no cost, whereas too tight a connection may leave you liable to pay extra. But don't expect anything more. You are not eligible for compensation for a missed connection.

✈ *Summary:* **At the Airport**

- Check for airport departure-tax requirements.

- Arrive in plenty of time.

- Get through to the lounge as soon as possible.

- Dress smartly, to improve chances of upgrades and get better customer service.

- Get the most you can if you are bumped owing to overbooking.

- Choose an aisle seat with extra legroom.

- Treat security seriously.

- Take particular care of your belongings at the security scanner.

- Make use of airline lounges if available.

- Allow enough time to get to the gate.

4 Beating Economy-Class Syndrome

With the airport scrum out of the way, it might seem that you can settle back and enjoy your flight. For the twenty-first-century flier, though, there is more to think about.

In a study published in January 2001 by Ashford Hospital, Surrey, the facility serving Heathrow Airport, it was revealed that at least one long-haul passenger dies of deep-vein thrombosis (DVT) each month within minutes of landing at the airport. Add in those whose symptoms develop later and those flying to other destinations and the picture is grim. Some estimates have put overall UK deaths as high as 2,000 a year. In the USA as many as 2 million people a year are said to have suffered from DVT to some degree.

DVT is the single biggest health concern for fliers at the start of the twenty-first century. The announcement that class-action lawsuits are now being prepared against a number of airlines will both ensure that much new evidence is forthcoming and keep the subject in the headlines for years to come.

Veins under pressure

For a long time the airlines have kept the risk suppressed as they packed seats in tighter and tighter to squeeze more passengers on to a plane. It shouldn't have been a surprise to them. The condition was pinpointed as a specific risk of flying over fifty years ago, when a doctor on a long flight from the USA to South America recognized the dangers. The same UK hospital that issued the 2001 report was pointing out as long ago as 1985 that passengers had a higher than normal tendency to some problems like embolisms (an artery blocked by a blood clot) shortly after landing from flights.

An analysis from Auckland, New Zealand, in the same year, 2001, showed a sixteen-fold increase in the likelihood of the reporting of a serious or life-threatening illness in the

---

Quick Tip: **Extra Risks**

Anyone over forty has an increased risk of deep-vein thrombosis, and this increases further in more elderly passengers. Both pregnancy and the contraceptive pill make it more likely that blood clots will form. There are also medical conditions that may increase risk: heart disease, cancer and the genetic condition Leiden V. If you are at increased risk, make sure that you take preventive action against DVT.

forty-eight hours following a long-haul flight. The statistics are frightening. In yet another study, on 100 susceptible fliers, published in November 2000, 10 per cent developed blood clots during a single flight. Many of these clots dissolve harmlessly, but any one could be fatal if it remained intact.

Deep-vein thrombosis caused by long-distance air travel was given the name 'economy-class syndrome' by I. S. Stack and B. H. R. Symington in 1977. Although this is in some ways a misleading label – it is perfectly possible to suffer from DVT when flying business or first class – it reflects some of the causes of this condition. It would help to be clear just what DVT is, though.

A thrombosis is the result of a blood clot – a small amount of blood that has solidified – being carried around the body to lodge in a dangerous and sometimes fatal location such as the lungs. Deep-vein thrombosis (DVT), so-called because it occurs in a deep, not a surface, vein usually in the calf or thigh, can occur when long-term pressure on a sensitive part of the body constricts a vein, making it easier for a clot to form. It isn't limited to air travellers by any means – anyone who stays in a relatively constant position with pressure on a limb has the potential to develop DVT, whether sitting in a long-distance coach or in front of a computer monitor. However, it is true that conditions on an aircraft make the risk greater – for example, a thrombosis is more likely to occur if the blood is thickened, a side effect of the thin air on board.

DVT is generally more of a risk for older passengers, but it can affect young, healthy fliers too. Much of the change in official reaction to DVT seems to have been triggered by the death of Emma Christoffersen, a healthy twenty-eight-year-old, who died after taking a Qantas flight from Sydney to London in October 2000.

Economy-class seating is particularly conducive to DVT, because the small amount of space provided makes it likely that you will sit in the same position for a long time. The seat edge will be pushed into your thighs. The reduced air pressure thickens the blood, making it easier for it to form a clot. Although more expensive seating gives you a better chance to avoid DVT, because you are not fixed in such a cramped, immobile position, it does have some dangers of its own – for instance, from badly designed leg-rests that may put pressure on the calves.

DVT is insidious because it does not necessarily have an immediate distressing effect. Initially there may be nothing at all. Most clots dissolve within a short time, but if the clot remains you are likely to develop swelling and pain in the leg, with a faint, bruise-like discolouration. This can occur days or even weeks after the flight. After this there are likely to be chest and shoulder pains as the clot reaches a danger point. Death can ensue very quickly after this.

Airborne aerobics

Exercise seems to be essential to minimize the risk of DVT. Try to move around the cabin at least once an hour. Realistically, though, this is often not practical, as the 'Fasten seat belts' signs can be left on for long periods and

Quick Tip: Chi Gung to the Rescue

The Chinese exercise regime of Chi Gung can be useful for working out in a limited space, even if you have no time for the philosophical trappings that accompany such disciplines. Chi Gung depends on focusing on specific movements and working against slow internal resistance. The following routine, devised for this book by a Chi Gung practitioner, can provide a good alternative approach to in-seat exercise.

- *Sit in an upright posture with your hands in your lap, your knees together, and your feet flat on the floor. Relax yourself by slowing your breathing and concentrating upon every breath, feeling the tension flow out with each exhalation.*

- *When you are relaxed, imagine that there is an incredibly heavy weight across your thighs. Slowly lift your heels, leaving your toes on the floor, all the while visualizing the resistance of this weight. Imagine while doing this that you are pushing your toes into the floor. Make the movement very slow.*

- *Now imagine that your knees are being held together. Slowly, and working against a huge resistance, separate them. Separate your heels at the same time as your knees (imagining the same resistance is in place against them), but keep your toes together. You need not spread your knees wide (even if the seat would allow it), but make the movement slow and hard work.*

- *Now imagine that your knees and heels are being held apart. Slowly, and working against a huge resistance, bring them together again.*

- *Slowly lower your heels to the floor, imagining that you have to squash something beneath them that is holding them away from the floor.*

- *Next, slowly lift your toes off the floor while keeping your heels firmly in place, imagining that the front parts of your feet are being held down by a huge resistance. Lower them again, fighting this resistance as you do so.*

- *Finally, concentrate on your buttocks. With every breath in, squeeze your buttocks together, taking as long to do this as the slow breath in takes to complete. Hold for a beat, and then as you slowly breathe out relax them, taking as long to complete the relaxation as the slow breath out takes. Repeat the buttock-squeezing a few times. (This has the added benefit of reducing the risk of getting piles that seems to accompany frequent flying.)*

- *Repeat the whole process until you are bored. If you intend to have a sleep on the flight, now would be a great time to have one.*

because the trolleys passing up and down cut off sections of the plane for what seems an age. Even so, you can make use of regular toilet breaks to keep you on the move without seeming too strange – and once in the toilet, really go to town, flexing and massaging your limbs with no fear of embarrassment. Even if you do have a workout every time you use the lavatory, it is worth getting some exercise in place in your seat as well. This can also help reduce the impact of jet lag.

Use a quick routine to ensure you reduce the risk of DVT and at the same time reduce stress. Start with your feet and work up your body (don't forget to go out to your fingertips), stretching and relaxing, rotating and flexing your body parts. This doesn't have to be anywhere near as embarrassingly obvious as it sounds – and, anyway, the amount of publicity DVT has received means that most people will be aware of the risks of not exercising. Go all the way up to the shoulders and neck. Take particular care to work the portions that are in contact with the seat or under pressure. Don't just move your thighs around, for instance – give them a gentle massage. This is quite possible without causing distress to nearby passengers.

Reducing the risk

While exercise is essential, it is not the only form of preventive action you can take. The simplest and most essential accompaniment to exercise is to keep drinking water and to hold off from alcohol, tea, coffee and other diuretics, which increase dehydration. As well as the benefits discussed when considering jet lag (see page 148), drinking plenty of water will ensure that dehydration does not make the impact of pressure on your legs worse. As a side effect, it will also force you to go to the toilet more often, making sure that you get enforced exercise.

If you do not have an adverse reaction to aspirin, taking a low dose (typically half an aspirin for an adult) has the effect of slightly thinning the blood and reducing the risk of clots. The ideal is to start a daily low dose three days before departure, but on the day is better than nothing. Make sure that this is acceptable to your GP.

Perhaps even more effective is the use of support stockings. These stop the pressure points having such an effect on the veins. They can be worn unobtrusively beneath trousers – it just requires a degree of fortitude to overcome the self-image problem that goes along with them.

Quick Tip: Good Support Takes Time

If you do decide to take the support-stocking route, note that most support stockings are made to order and will take a day or two to arrive, so it is best to visit the chemist well in advance.

It makes a lot of sense to take such precautions, but, just as those seeking to slim should not rely on diet alone, don't forget to exercise. It is much better to combine exercise with other precautions than to rely on the precautions alone.

Is it really economy-class syndrome?

Underlying the popular name for the condition, 'economy-class syndrome', is the implication that DVT is a problem peculiar to those travelling cheap. While this certainly isn't true – there are well-documented cases of travellers in other classes suffering from DVT – it is true that travelling in economy does increase the chances of suffering from DVT, as do other factors like age, tendency to heart disease, and pregnancy.

The cramped seated position in economy, with very limited legroom and the lack of support for the lower legs, putting extra pressure on the thighs, makes it more difficult to counter the conditions that encourage the onset of DVT. In a business-class or first-class seat it is much easier to stretch out and perform in-seat exercises, and there will be some leg support (though this can put pressure on other parts of the leg).

Perhaps the benefits of premium seating will be felt most when you decide to sleep during flights. Premium seats usually provide a much flatter sleeping surface. Also, there is room to turn on to your side if this is your natural sleeping position. This makes it more likely that you will undergo the natural in-sleep motions that tend to be prevented by sleeping seated upright. It is hard to justify paying the extra that airlines charge for business class (unless someone else is paying for you), but there is no doubt that you are buying extra legroom, particularly on long-haul flights. Those more expensive seats will be tipping the scales in your favour.

If you can't run to business-class fares, bear in mind that the distance between economy-class seats does vary from airline to airline. At the time of writing, the charter companies and some smaller airlines (carriers like Airtours, Air 2000, Britannia and JMC) were offering the worst seating, with an evil pitch of 28 inches. This means that anyone over 1.75 m (5 foot 10 inches) tall – around the average height for men – is going to have his or her legs crammed into the seat in front. The opportunities for motion become almost zero, while the number of pressure points is increased.

Quick Tip: **Pitching a Seat**

The figures given for seat pitch are invariably in inches, as US standards dominate the engineering side of the airline business. Twenty-eight inches corresponds to 70 cm, 32 inches to 80 cm and 36 inches to 90 cm.

Note that seat pitch does not describe the amount of legroom (if only!). It refers to the length of cabin occupied by the seat and the legroom combined – that's to say, the distance between the same position on two seats.

It seems amazing that airlines can offer such cramped seating, especially as the average passenger has been increasing in size each year. But the legal recommended minimum is even smaller – a ridiculous 26 inches, which the Civil Aviation Authority deems is capable of being escaped from in an emergency by most passengers. Most of the well-known airlines are at present somewhere in the range between 30 and 32 inches (Air France, British Airways, British Midland, United, Virgin and others). Particularly promising were Air New Zealand, Alitalia and some Cathay Pacific flights, which reached 33 inches.

Way out in front is American Airlines, which on some aircraft has got as far as 36 inches. This is because American has consciously taken out 7 per cent of the seating in economy as a direct response to the customer outcry over DVT. We can expect to see other airlines follow suit, and hopefully the more comfortable 36 inches will become the norm. Check the seat pitch with your airline before booking (particularly if you are tall). But bear in mind that it takes time to put a whole fleet of aircraft through a refit. Just because an airline says that it is 'changing its seating configuration' doesn't mean that it will have got as far as the plane you fly on at a particular date.

DVT in proportion

DVT is a real threat. But we do need to keep the risk in proportion. Even without taking any precautions against DVT, the vast majority of travellers do not have any problems after a long-haul flight. However, now we know what we are dealing with, it would be very unwise to avoid the opportunities to lower the risk.

✈ *Summary:* Beating Economy-Class Syndrome

- Deep Vein Thrombosis (DVT) is encouraged when sustained pressure on a sensitive part of the body constricts a vein.

- Regular exercise and massaging of affected parts when on board will help significantly.

- Dehydration is also a factor – drink plenty of bottled water and avoid diuretics (alcohol, coffee, tea, cola).

- Supplementary preventatives (aspirin, support stockings) are recommended.

- DVT is not limited to economy-class travellers.

5 Hypoxia – Breathing with Altitude

Air is something we take for granted, but one of the incidental effects of being pushed up nearly a dozen kilometres into the sky is that the atmosphere outside the plane bears no resemblance to the air we breathe at ground level. Think of the precautions that a climber facing Mount Everest takes. He or she faces a hugely hostile environment, yet it is less harsh than the conditions outside the aircraft window. The human body was no more designed to operate in such an environment than it was to exist on the surface of the moon.

A hostile environment

It's a simple fact that air pressure drops with altitude. By the time you reach 68,000 ft (around 20 km up – but aircraft altitudes are still measured in feet) the air pressure is practically zero. Breathing is impossible. Blood boils. Yet supersonic aircraft like Concorde fly near this, at 60,000 ft (18 km), and even at a conventional airliner's cruising height of 37,000 ft (11 km) there is no hope of surviving an exposure of more than a few seconds.

If it is so unpleasant, why fly so high? The answer is a combination of economics and safety. The higher a plane flies, the less resistance the air offers – and that means a reduction in expenditure on fuel, the single largest non-human expense for any airline. Equally, if an aircraft encounters serious problems, the height gives a measure of time to sort them out before the aircraft hits the ground. Also, by flying at this sort of height the plane is above the weather. Most storms cannot reach it, and that means much less of the airsickness that was a common feature of early air travel when planes couldn't reach such an altitude.

Yet there is a price to pay for pushing up towards the edge of space. The aircraft cabin needs to be kept pressurized, pumped up like a rigid balloon to ensure that the people inside can breathe. In principle, this pressure could be made that of ground level, but the greater the pressure the more risk there is of leaking, and the more need to strengthen the aircraft, and that means more weight and more cost. When pressurization was first considered, an air pressure equivalent to an arbitrary maximum altitude of around 8,000 ft (2,400 m) was set as the comfort level. To this day, most aircraft cabins are set at a pressure equivalent to between 6,000 and 8,000 ft. Concorde is one of the few planes where considerable design effort was put into making the environment better for passengers: it was decided to keep the equivalent pressure down to 5,000 ft, to improve the pilots' night vision (see below) and to reduce stress both on the crew and on the high-fare-paying passengers.

The standard pressure level was not devised using any

scientific testing, but seems to have been based on the maximum height at which there are a significant number of populated areas around the world. (Mexico City, for example, lies at 7,500 ft.) However, there is a problem that comes with altitude. As the air pressure decreases, the amount of oxygen available to breath drops too. At typical cabin pressure there is between 20 and 26 per cent less oxygen for the passengers than there is at sea level. And too little oxygen leads to a potentially dangerous condition – hypoxia: a deficiency in the amount of oxygen that reaches body tissues.

Flying on thin air

For a normal passenger, the result of the level of hypoxia induced by normal cabin air pressure will be only a slight increase in the rate of the heartbeat and breathing. Night vision will become slightly impaired. Fatigue levels will rise, and the ability to learn will fall. However, some common chronic diseases already cut down the amount of oxygen that is received at a normal altitude. With the extra reduction caused by the cabin pressure, there is a real danger of triggering serious problems.

Sufferers from heart, lung and blood-vessel diseases in particular will find that, along with chronic-bronchitis sufferers and others, they may need extra oxygen to cope with the effect of the cabin pressure. See the table on page 361 for suggested diseases where it would be wise to consult a doctor before travelling. It is also worth noting that some medications will become more or less effective under lower air pressure and under the stress of flying. Epileptics may be more liable to attack and have to increase levels of medication. There is some evidence that insulin-using diabetics have had to increase dosage when travelling westbound and decrease it when travelling to the east. Again, consult your GP.

For the rest of us, the biggest implication is probably the increased fatigue level and the decreased ability to learn. Travelling at around 8,000 feet practically doubles the rate at which you become tired, making it easy to feel shattered after a long flight. (In fact this is a major contributor to jet lag.) Concentrating on anything from business papers to a demanding book takes significantly more effort.

Making it worse

The impact of hypoxia is arguably just as much a justification for the sustained banning of smoking on aircraft as are passive smoking and the increased fire risk. Like most products from burning carbon, cigarette smoke contains a percentage of the dangerous substance carbon monoxide (the gas that causes death when car exhaust fumes are breathed). One of the effects of carbon monoxide on the body is to reduce the amount of oxygen reaching the blood. In effect, smoking a cigarette on board has the result of increasing your apparent altitude from (say) 6,000 feet to 12,000, with the associated increased levels of hypoxia. This means more fatigue, less concentration, and an increased risk to those who are susceptible to conditions aggravated by hypoxia.

Smoking has been banned on many flights, but some carriers do still allow it, particularly on long-haul routes. If you have a choice, see if you can get on a non-smoking carrier. If you can't, try to make sure that you are near the middle of the non-smoking section (there will probably be a business-class or first-class smoking section in front of you). A sneaky way to avoid smoke if you are really suffering is to ask for a portable oxygen bottle because you are having trouble breathing. The crew will have to stop all smoking for three rows on either side of you while you are using it. There is no smoking allowed in the toilets either, so they provide a temporary haven.

If you are smoker, you may feel aggrieved that you are being prevented from smoking, and there is some evidence that being made to avoid smoking during long journeys can be a contributory factor to air rage. If you can't face a long flight without a cigarette, look at ways of making your journey in shorter hops. Alternatively, try nicotine-delivery methods like gum and patches. It's quite surprising that airlines don't offer these as a matter of course, if only to reduce the risk of air rage. But the combination of the effect that smoking will have on your own hypoxia with the very serious fire risk and the inevitable heavy dose of passive smoking passed on to others may just persuade you that, in the air at least, you can temporarily give up tobacco.

It is probable but not certain that alcohol has a similar effect to breathing smoke, again reducing the amount of oxygen that manages to get through to the bloodstream and hence increasing the impact of hypoxia. It is certainly true that the effect of alcoholic drinks at high altitude is subjectively greater, which when combined with the dehydrating impact of alcohol makes them best avoided altogether.

In the unlikely event...

For most travellers, the effects of limited oxygen are an irritant but nothing more. However, a few will at some point in their flying life encounter decompression, the situation where the plane's protective mechanisms fail and the cabin pressure drops below the normal. This can happen dramatically – so-called explosive decompression, where perhaps a window blows out and the pressure plummets towards the outside level – but more often it comes about in an insidious way as pressure slowly falls.

Such a gradual decompression won't catch the pilot by surprise. As pressure levels drop to the equivalent of 10,000 ft, the pilot receives a warning and will take the plane down to a lower altitude. This is very necessary – prolonged exposure to the pressure at between 15,000 and 20,000 ft can result in physical or mental impairment, and anything above 20,000 ft will lead to unconsciousness and death.

Depressurization is uncommon. It is highly unlikely to happen on your next flight. But it is worth being aware that it is not confined to Hollywood dramas. In the ten-year period from 1974 to 1983 there were 355 depressurization incidents on US commercial flights. Of these, around

150 – 15 per year – were serious enough for oxygen masks to deploy or for there to be injury.

When the cabin pressure level exceeds around 10,000 feet, oxygen masks should drop from the ceiling, as is shown in every pre-flight demonstration. If this should happen, it is important to make use of the masks. If there is a gradual depressurization, one of the effects of the slow drop in the cabin pressure is that the occupants feel a 'high' not unlike the impact of alcohol. This can lead to an artificial sense of security, making the passengers feel that there is nothing wrong and that the masks have dropped accidentally. In many incidents nearly half the passengers don't bother to use the masks. But lack of oxygen is a serious risk – assume that the worst has happened until the crew tell you otherwise. If your mask doesn't drop down, find one over an empty seat, or ask the cabin crew for an oxygen cylinder.

With the mask dangling before you, pull it towards you – the tug on the attached 'lanyard' (piece of string) will start the oxygen flowing. In some more modern aircraft, instead of the mask a streamer drops down. Pulling on this both drops the mask and starts the air supply, making it easier to make sure you will be able to breathe as soon as the mask is over your face. Pull the elastic band over your head to hold the mask in place, and breath as normally as you can in such circumstances.

In the safety briefing, you will probably hear the instruction to get your mask on before looking after your children (or anyone else). At face value this is an unpleasant or even an unnatural instruction. We all want to keep our children safe, and might tend to put them first despite what the briefing says. But (though unfortunately most briefings don't explain why) it is essential to follow these instructions.

If the cabin air pressure drops so much that you go over the equivalent of 20,000 ft, you will have only a brief time, perhaps fifteen seconds of consciousness, to get your mask on. Once it is on, you have still got time to get the mask on your child or children, as even if they have already passed out there will still be precious seconds before permanent damage ensues. But if you spend the few seconds during which you are still capable of taking action looking after your child, you may well then end up unconscious with no one to give you assistance with that essential oxygen.

Explosive decompression

In the event of explosive decompression, it is very obvious that things have gone wrong. There will be a loud bang. It is not unusual for one or more people near the hole (if it is visible) to be sucked out of the aircraft with the first dramatic rush of air, even if they have their seatbelts fastened. The aircraft will probably be in a nose-down position as the pilot rapidly loses height. Here it is even more important to get to your oxygen supply as quickly as possible. Thrown forward in your seat, you may be tempted to push your face into the mask. Don't – remember, it is necessary to pull it towards you to start the oxygen supply. Even if you can't sit back in your seat and need to pull the mask past your head first, make sure you pull back on it before starting to use it.

If such a depressurization happens while the plane is halfway across the Atlantic, the pilot has another problem to face. Although he or she will initially drop the plane to perhaps 10,000 ft, once the situation is under control it is impossible to stay there. A typical airliner does not carry enough fuel to complete the journey in the face of such increased air resistance. To get by, the plane will usually have to return to between 15,000 and 20,000 ft. And, though every plane carries enough oxygen to provide for everyone's needs during the initial emergency, there will not be enough on board for everyone to use throughout the journey.

Typically, between 15 and 30 per cent of the passengers will be able to continue breathing extra oxygen all the way home. This will make for an uncomfortable flight for the rest, as the reduced oxygen levels will make the majority of the passengers without masks act as if they are drunk. These passengers have to suffer the results of prolonged exposure to a high altitude. In the very unlikely event that this happens to you, it is essential to get a check-up from a qualified aviation-medicine expert after the event. Don't assume that everything is all right just because you feel OK when you get off the plane – problems due to oxygen deficiency can take a considerable time to surface.

Panic attacks

According to the American Medical Association, the most
common medical condition that occurs on board aircraft is
another problem that results from a decreased level of gas
intake, but in this case the gas is carbon dioxide. Although
we don't need carbon dioxide in order to live, the body
monitors carbon-dioxide levels as part of its balancing
system. If the levels drop, the body's response is to push up
the breathing rate. But, as there is often nothing to compensate for, the result is overbreathing – hyperventilation –
sometimes described as a panic attack.

Not only does the lower air pressure on board mean a
slightly lower level of carbon dioxide in the air, hence an
increased risk of hyperventilation, there is also a close link
between hyperventilation and stress, for which the combination of fear and excitement that usually accompanies
flight provides a ready trigger. Then the poor victim is into
a vicious circle. The results of hyperventilation can be quite
frightening and so trigger more anxiety, raising the level of
hyperventilation.

One of the reasons why this body reaction is so frightening is that it has significant similarities to the impact of a
heart attack. There is breathlessness, and often numbness
and tingling in the limbs. There can be palpitations, muscle
spasms and blurred vision. The person looks grey and
seriously ill. This often leads to mistaken medical call-outs
on the ground, and can trigger panic in the environment of
an aircraft cabin without proper medical support. What's

more, the extra oxygen that would be given to help those with heart or breathing troubles will make hyperventilation not better but worse.

In fact the cure is dramatically simple. We exhale much more carbon dioxide than there is present in the air normally, so simply by rebreathing your own exhaled breath it is possible to overcome the effects of hyperventilation in a minute or two. The easiest way to do this is to place a paper bag (never plastic, due to the dangers of asphyxiation) over the mouth and nose and try to breathe normally. The airline's sickbags are perfectly good for this operation.

Ears a-poppin'

There is one last problem that can arise from changes in cabin air pressure. As the pressure decreases, pockets of air trapped in parts of the body will expand. The most obvious example of this is in the middle ear, where some air is almost always trapped by the twisted Eustachian tube that links it to the mouth and nose. This results in the typical popping sensation as the eardrum on the outside of the middle ear reverberates to the displacement of air. It also can result in considerable discomfort if the air pressure cannot be equalized between the middle ear and the aircraft cabin.

Usually it is enough to swallow or yawn to encourage the air through the tube, but, if this fails, uneven pressure can usually be overcome by holding the nose closed, closing the mouth, and blowing gently down the nose (a technique that delights in the name of the Valsalva manoeuvre). If you are suffering from a bad cold or an allergic reaction, the Eustachian tube could be swollen or partly blocked, which will make it harder to equalize the pressure. This particularly affects children, whose smaller tubes block more easily, and at the extreme can result in burst eardrums. Ideally, children with bad head colds and similar infections should not fly.

Similarly, blocked sinuses can result in a considerable amount of pain as pressure levels change. Having some form of nasal decongestant can help, but serious sinus problems may result in injury, so this is another condition where it is worth checking with your GP before flight.

If you can't unblock either the ears or the sinuses and the pain continues, it is worth resorting to a remedy similar to that used in dealing with the childhood complaint called croup. Croup is, in effect, laryngitis, but in the child's smaller airways the inflammation results in much more discomfort, accompanied by strange, barking gulps for breath. The ideal solution for croup is cool steam, as both cool air and the moisture content of steam quickly help to soothe and reduce the swelling. Exactly the same approach can be taken with ear and sinus problems.

Quick Tip: **Steaming at the Ears**

Getting a source of (cool) steam to relieve pressure on the ear or nose is not particularly easy on an aircraft. The best approach is to put some paper towels in the bottom of a cup, soaking them in hot water from the galley, then pour off the water and hold your ear or nose over the cup. Whatever you do, don't get hot water in your ear or up your nose though.

Under pressure

The tendency to expand as pressure falls is not limited to the natural air pockets in the body. All gases expand as confining pressure decreases. This makes it best to avoid food that is liable to generate wind, as there is an increased risk of stomach pains. More significant, though, is the presence of nitrogen in the blood of scuba divers.

All divers know that it is necessary to return to the surface slowly after a deep dive, as the nitrogen in the breathing mixture will have been forced into the blood and tissues. As it comes back out, it forms tiny bubbles which if released too quickly result in the agonizing and dangerous condition called the bends. What fewer divers know is that this condition will be exacerbated by the low cabin pressure on an airliner. The American Medical Association suggests leaving a minimum of 12 hours after any dive before flying, and 24 hours after any dive over 10 m in depth.

There are also occasional opportunities for artificial air pockets to form, usually after some form of medical treatment. When a broken limb is protected in a plaster cast, it is quite possible for pockets of air to develop between the cast and the limb. A combination of a swollen limb and the attempt of these air pockets to expand can be dangerous. In 1982 a twelve-year-old boy was travelling on a seven-hour flight from Canada to South America with his legs in plaster. By the time he arrived his legs had become gangrenous. As it is not uncommon to pick up a plaster cast on a skiing holiday or from a motoring accident abroad, make sure that the cast is professionally split before undertaking a flight, particularly when travelling long-haul.

Similarly, when you undergo surgery – or, for that matter, suffer a cut or serious scrape of any form – air is introduced into the wound. For a serious wound this can take anything between a week and a month to be properly reabsorbed. If exposed to the low pressure of the cabin, the trapped air can expand and cause a haemorrhage. If you have any doubt, consult your doctor before flying after an operation or with a major wound.

✈ *Summary:* Hypoxia – Breathing with Altitude

- The air pressure in an aircraft cabin is equivalent to that around 8,000 ft (2,400 m) up a mountain.

- In-flight air has between 20 and 26 per cent less oxygen than at sea level.

- Sufferers from heart, lung and blood-vessel diseases need to be particularly wary of the effects of hypoxia.

- Hypoxia results in an increased rate of fatigue and an increased difficulty when trying to study.

- Smoking will add the equivalent of another 6,000 ft to the reduction in oxygen levels experienced.

- If oxygen masks are deployed, make sure you pull yours towards you.

- Always fit your own mask before helping anyone else.

- If a plane is depressurized in mid-flight and has to return to 15–20,000 ft to complete the journey, ensure that you are checked by a specialist after the flight.

- Hyperventilation can be cured by breathing into a paper bag. Don't use oxygen.

- If necessary, try cool steam to help release pressure in the ears or sinuses.

- Divers should wait 12 to 24 hours between their last dive and flying.

- Plaster casts should be loosened professionally before flying.

6 Sick-Aircraft Syndrome

A lack of oxygen isn't the only potential problem with the air in flight. As much as half the air on board at any one time has been recycled. This gives rise to a potential health risk, compounding the danger of infection from occupants of nearby seats. The cabin air can spread anything from a cold to life-threatening diseases – a particular concern is the spread of tuberculosis. Many people also suffer from regular minor illness after flying, as the dry air reduces the effectiveness of the nasal membranes and increases the chances of infection.

Add to this the possibility of a negative reaction to the insecticide sprays still common on some routes, and increasing concerns of air pollution from toxic industrial chemicals used in aircraft engineering, and the air on board smells anything but sweet.

Flying in the Sahara

The absence of one, simple substance has the most consistent impact on the air traveller. That substance is water.

The air inside a plane is incredibly dry, and as a result will have an impact on your skin, your eyes and more.

Quick Tip: Get Moist

Aircraft cabin air is so dry that it has as low as 1 per cent relative humidity. Compare this to the 30 to 65 per cent that the National Institute for Occupational Safety and Health considers as the comfort zone. This extreme dryness makes it easier for germs to spread. By using a water spray to keep your nasal membranes moist and by drinking lots of fluids – experts recommend a glass of water an hour – you can reduce the impact of the dry air.

To put the dryness of cabin air in context, a typical damp day outdoors in the UK reaches about 80 per cent relative humidity. Indoors, with high-efficiency air conditioning, this falls to as low as 25 per cent. But this is a tropical humidity compared with the air provided on airliners once they are at cruising height. Humidity levels on board will start at around the air-conditioned 25 per cent mark. Once the aircraft is aloft, the air entering the cabin has practically no moisture in it. It is only the water vapour produced by the passengers that keeps levels up, but gradually the humidity will slip away, tending towards the 1 per cent level.

The dehydration from this dryness creeps up on you. You don't sweat, as you would in the hot sun, nor do you feel thirsty. And this dryness doesn't just make it easier for infection to spread. Eyes, nose, throat and skin all begin to feel uncomfortable. Those who suffer from eczema and other dry-skin problems will find their conditions getting worse.

While a water spray is great for the nasal membranes, water is not so good for the skin, as it mostly evaporates and is wasted. It is better to use a rehydrating gel or a moisturiser. As an alternative to the spray, breathe through a water-soaked handkerchief (which may slightly cut down on the chances of picking up an air-transmitted disease too) – though this is inconvenient over a long flight. If you wear contact lenses, take them out or regularly soak them in fluid during the flight.

As well as increasing your fluid intake, it is worth avoiding diuretics – substances that increase the amount of liquid you lose when you pass water. The usual problem drinks are anything alcoholic, coffee, tea and colas.

→ Fast Track:
Controlling Dehydration

• Use a moistened handkerchief to increase the humidity of the air you breathe.

• Drink at least a glass of bottled water an hour.

• Avoid diuretics like alcohol, coffee, tea and colas.

• Remove contact lenses.

Stale air

The cabin air supply may be dry, but it seems reasonable to assume that air from high in the sky has not suffered too much from human pollution. Unfortunately, however, the outside air is not the only source of gases that passengers breathe. Up to 50 per cent of the air entering the cabin through the vents has been recirculated after passing through filters. The remainder comes in through the engines, after having been cooled and filtered. The amount of this 'fresh' air you receive varies considerably according to where you sit. According to a 1986 US report on aircraft cabin air, first- and business-class travellers receive between two and three times as much fresh air per person as those in economy.

In fact it can be worse than this. In a 747, the flight crew get between 60 and 150 cu. ft of air per minute, first-class passengers between 30 and 50 cu. ft per minute, and economy as little as 7. While flight crew are provided with a separate air supply, the better conditions for first-class and business passengers reflect the fact that fewer breathing bodies are packed into the space. The air also tends to flow from the front of the aircraft to the back, becoming less fresh as it goes. The remarkably low economy figure of 7 cu. ft per minute compares badly with the 20 cu. ft per minute minimum recommended by the American Society of Heating, Refrigeration and Air Conditioning Engineers (ASHRAE).

Why isn't more fresh air used? The reason, as with the altitude flown at, is primarily one of cost. A 747 has three air-conditioning packs, one of which is usually kept switched off. In an experiment undertaken by the plane manufacturer McDonnell Douglas it was found that each aircraft can save around 70,000 gallons of fuel a year by keeping the recirculation rate up. But in terms of cost to the individual passenger for a flight the cost is trivial. On a full 747 it would cost around 12p per passenger per hour to keep the extra air-conditioning pack in operation.

It may well be worth the airlines raising the ventilation rate and using it as a selling point. Otherwise this saving is reminiscent of the time when a major airline decided to save money by stopping automatically giving out nuts with drinks in first class. As the complaints started to come in, it was realized that a single first-class frequent flier more than paid for every nut that was used in a year. The nuts were reinstated.

While the effects of low pressure are very clearly documented, it is less clear just what, if anything, this low volume of fresh air does to the passenger. There is some subjective evidence that it can make the effects of hypoxia worse and encourage the onset of hyperventilation. So, if you do seem to be suffering from some combination of excessive fatigue, the inability to concentrate, accelerated heart rate, breathlessness, numbness, clammy skin and a headache, it is worth asking the cabin crew if they could ask the captain to turn on all the air packs and cut the recirculating fans, as you are having trouble breathing. This could be referred to as 'full utilization' or 'engaging all the environmental control units' or similar jargon, depending on the plane manufacturer and the nationality of the aircrew. If things don't get better, ask for one of the portable oxygen bottles, explaining that you are finding it difficult to breath (but remember that hyperventilation is made worse, not better, by extra oxygen).

Airlines will point out that the linkage of air recycling and the financial bottom line is not quite so obvious as clean-air campaigners suggest. They say that recirculation is not just used to save money, but is also a mechanism to increase cabin humidity. It is certainly true that higher humidity is a side effect of recirculation, but there are other and better ways to obtain this without allowing stale and possibly infected and tainted air to be returned to the cabin.

The bad-air jet

In October 2000 a committee of the Australian parliament was requested by the senate to report on the air quality in the popular short-range passenger jet the BAe 146. The resulting report was unusual in its detailed consideration of the problems of bad cabin air, and made it clear that, while the committee concentrated on the BAe 146, the problems they found were common in many other aircraft.

The 146 has a reputation for having a 'smelly' cabin, and it was this, coupled with occupational-health concerns from crew, that had triggered the investigation. As the non-technical members of the committee soon discovered, there is only one place that air can sensibly come from at the altitude at which an aircraft flies – the engines, in which the air is brought up to a high pressure. Generally there is no fuel in this air, as it comes out of the engine before it reaches the chamber where combustion takes place. But there is a possibility of getting compressor oil and other contaminants in the air if an oil leak takes place, and the 146 seemed more susceptible than most to leaks of the oil.

The committee noted that ASHRAE was developing a standard to ensure that cabin air quality is safe, minimizes the potential of adverse health effects, and is comfortable for the occupants. At the time of writing, this standard is yet to be firmed up – a lack of urgency that perhaps reflects the outcome of a February 2001 ASHRAE report suggesting that air-contaminant levels in most aircraft were significantly lower than those in residential and commercial buildings. However, the report's authors did note that they were dealing with only a very small sample (three aircraft types on ten flights) and would need more information before they could make more conclusive remarks.

In a submission to the Australian government committee, Dr Jean Christophe Balouet noted that about 70 smoke events and 500 serious fume events, affecting around 40,000 passengers and crew, take place worldwide each year. Symptoms from fumes described to the committee included dizziness, nausea, vomiting, headaches, numbing, breathing difficulties, and irritation to eyes, nose and throat. Often these problems seemed linked to leaking jet-engine oil – in many cases to a synthetic material, Mobil Jet Oil II. This contains tricresyl phosphate, classified by the Australian National Industrial Chemicals Notification and Assessment Scheme as toxic.

Chromosome analysis of a number of BAe 146 crew revealed evidence of exposure to 'significant levels of chemical toxins, sufficient to cause grave, short and long term health consequences'. Although claiming not to be influenced by reports of toxicity, Mobil told the committee that it was developing a new oil with less toxic additives.

The committee finally recommended introducing a national standard for checking and monitoring engine seals and air quality in commercial jets. It also asked for specific procedures for the 146 to ensure that faulty aircraft were withdrawn from service, that sources of contamination be identified and further evaluated, and that an 'appropriate and accurate' test be developed to detect the presence of chemical fumes in aircraft cabins. There was also a request to set up a study into the effects of aircraft-cabin air on passengers and crew – an activity that has not been undertaken in any detail since an inconclusive 1986 US report. Finally, there was a proposal to assess how quickly high-grade air filters could be fitted to minimize contamination.

Engine oil isn't the only problem that such filters have to deal with. Toxic chemical vapours can originate from hydraulic spills and from aviation fuel laced with pesticide additives to kill fungus and algae. Thousands of complaints have been filed by Alaska Air flight attendants alone. Recently, twenty-six Alaska Air flight attendants filed a class-action lawsuit, blaming the hydraulic fluid Skydrol, described by environmental-health specialist George Ewing MD as a neurotoxin, for adverse effects on their health. The problem now involves many airlines and many types of aircraft, compounding the concern about cabin air quality. Following on from the Australian parliamentary inquiry, similar investigations are under way on behalf of the US National Institute of Occupational Safety and Health and the UK House of Lords Subcommittee on Science and Technology. Cabin air quality is set to be a major battleground during the next few years.

Quick Tip: **The Cover-Up**

Unless you are prepared to use a proper filter mask (see page 126), the only real option to deal with cabin air pollution is to improvise. In the days when dusty roads made travel on horseback and in carriages unpleasant it was common to use a kerchief to keep the dust out of the mouth and nose. A large enough handkerchief makes a good modern equivalent. But, to give it a chance of picking up the smaller pollutants, soak it in (bottled) water first.

As a positive side effect, this will also increase the humidity of the air you breathe, helping to reduce the dehydrating effect of bone-dry cabin air.

Every breath you take

According to the US Federal Center for Disease Control, an infectious or contagious disease (like flu) can easily spread through more than 70 per cent of the passengers on board during a flight. In a sealed aircraft with up to half its air recirculated there is plenty of opportunity for spreading disease, and, though cabin air is quite stringently filtered, there is a particularly strong risk from those sitting in close proximity to you for a long period of time.

Mostly the risk is of catching common infections like colds – most frequent fliers seem to suffer considerably more of these than the rest of the population – but there have been clearly identified cases where dangerous diseases have been spread around the cabin, most worryingly tuberculosis. There is a strong psychological difficulty in wearing a filter mask, but it certainly will cut down your chances of being infected.

Quick Tip: Masking the Problem

Masks, costing between £10 and £30, are available that will cut out around 98 per cent of airborne infections. The smaller masks are not dissimilar to those used by dentists and workers in dusty environments – not too obtrusive to wear, but definitely liable to get you some strange looks. The Aviation Health Institute (see page 328) sells a range of masks.

If you can't face a mask, you may be able to cut down the chance of infection a little by using a nasal spray of water to keep the nasal membranes effective (don't drown yourself!) and then applying a small amount of edible oil to the inside of the nostrils. This is supposed to reduce the chances of infection getting in through cracks in the nasal skin. Wash your hands first, though, or you will do more harm than good.

→ Fast Track:
Avoiding Infection

- Consider buying a mask.

- Use a moistened handkerchief as a makeshift mask.

- Use a nasal spray of water to keep membranes moist.

- Use an edible oil on the insides of the nostrils to cover skin cracks.

- Ensure that your immunizations are up to date.

The ozone lie

Even if every aircraft had perfect protection from disease and the toxic chemicals introduced by the airline, there would still be one poison all around the plane as it glided through the air. The offending substance is ozone.

Generally speaking, ozone has a misleadingly good press. It's the useful stuff that forms a protective layer in the upper atmosphere, preventing us all from frying in ultra-violet radiation. And it tends to be associated with the healthy smells of seaweed and brine on the beach. In fact, though, as far as breathing it goes, ozone is an unpleasant poison. A US House of Representatives Hearing report of 1979, *Adverse Health Effects of Inflight Exposure to Atmospheric Ozone*, states that repeated exposure to ozone can lead to permanent lung scarring and loss of lung function. Ozone is related to the oxygen we breathe, but it is formed of molecules containing three oxygen atoms instead of two, making it entirely different chemically. The association with the seaside is spurious too – ozone is more the smell of electrical discharge and overworked laser printers than the fresh air of the beach.

The higher an aircraft flies, the greater the presence of ozone. Over around 45,000 ft there is a particularly sharp increase in concentration. Up at the 60,000-ft altitude that supersonic aircraft like Concorde fly at, ozone levels can be around 6 parts per million. This doesn't sound much, but is 60 times higher than the recommended maximum dosage. Concorde has platinum-based catalytic converters that break up the ozone and turn it into harmless oxygen, but these depend on the heat of the engine for their operation. This means that at the start of a descent, when Concorde is still high but the engines have been throttled back, cabin ozone levels rise by up to a factor of three. This isn't enough to be too concerned about during the couple of minutes or so when levels go up, but it does increase exposure.

It is also true that the catalytic converters of all airliners can be suspect. A 1994 Harvard survey of aircraft cabins found that as many as 20 per cent of trips were taken with converters that were working sufficiently poorly for unacceptable levels of ozone to get through. A pollutant like ozone that is very similar to the air we breathe is difficult to remove without the use of a catalytic converter. Breathing through a dampened handkerchief will reduce ozone levels slightly, as ozone tends to react with the water, but some will get through. Beyond this, there is little more the passenger can do other than lobby politicians for improved standards.

Beating the bugs

The attempt to control insects also raises concerns among passengers. The reasoning behind the pest control is excellent. Aircraft, like restaurant kitchens, are excellent breeding grounds for pests like cockroaches, and a wide range of undesirable insects can come aboard a plane when the cabin doors are open, then be transported to another country where they can spread disease to both people and crops.

Unfortunately there is no effective way to kill off insects which hasn't also got some dubious side effects for humans. Either one-shot insecticide is sprayed in the cabin during flight or on landing, or long-lasting chemicals are used to treat the aircraft every few weeks. Practically every chemical used in these processes has some hazardous qualities, but there is little you can do to avoid skin contact. However, you can at least reduce the impact of breathing the sprays by wearing a mask or breathing through a moistened handkerchief.

If you want to prevent yourself from being sprayed and are a sufferer from a complaint like asthma that may be aggravated by the spray, or are pregnant, you can get a certificate of exemption. This doesn't stop the plane being sprayed: it just means you are allowed to cover yourself up as much as you can manage in order to avoid contact with the spray. Where the spray is undertaken after landing, you may be allowed off the plane first (though there is no guarantee of this). Warn the cabin crew if you have a certificate, so that they can give you some advance warning to prepare. Make sure you have your respirator if you are likely to need one. Unfortunately the airline's oxygen bottles won't be suitable here, as their masks have little holes in them to balance air pressure and so won't protect you.

→ Fast Track:
Beating the Bugs

• Wear a mask or breathe through a moistened handkerchief.

• If you are pregnant or suffer from a breathing complaint, get a certificate of exemption from your doctor.

• If you use a respirator, make sure you have it handy.

• Have a shower as soon as possible, to rinse off any insecticide still on your skin.

Whether or not you suffer from a potentially affected condition, it is a good idea to have a shower as soon as possible after getting off the plane, to minimize the absorption of the pesticide through the skin. If the airline uses the residual method, where the cabin is permanently soaked with a 'background' insecticide, it is a good move to wear long clothing (just as it is for protection in the event of a crash), to reduce the amount of direct contact your skin makes with the treated surfaces in the cabin.

✈ *Summary:* Sick-Aircraft Syndrome

- Cabin air can be polluted and infected. It will certainly be extremely dry.

- Consider buying a mask, or using a moistened handkerchief to act as a mask.

- Drink plenty of bottled water, and avoid alcohol, coffee, tea and colas.

- If you are having difficulty breathing, ask for the cabin air to be turned up to full utilization.

- Ask for an oxygen bottle if you are still having trouble breathing (but not if you are hyperventilating – see page 111).

- Consider paying extra to fly in business or first class and get better quality air.

7 Bad Vibes

Few frequent fliers are aware that by regularly taking to the skies they are significantly increasing their exposure to life-threatening cosmic radiation. This consists of intense electromagnetic rays, like high-power X-rays, that bombard the earth from outside our solar system. The sun, too, pours out a wide band of radiation, and brings a dramatically increased risk when sunspots flare up. Such radiation is usually screened out by the atmosphere, but how much more dangerous is it when flying high on a plane? It is hard not to be concerned when it turns out that an average trip across the Atlantic exposes the traveller to as much radiation as a chest X-ray.

A real risk

For years now there have been scare stories about the dangers of using mobile phones or living near high-voltage power cables. In these examples of electromagnetic radiation there is little hard evidence of risk. The latest report in 2001 concluded that any linkage that existed was very weak. The impact of natural radiation and the way travelling by air makes it worse is a different matter. This is not something concocted by public panic or scaremongering: it is solid, substantiated fact.

According to the National Radiological Protection Board (NRPB), the UK's independent body dealing with radiation exposure, 'it is assumed that however low the dose, there is some risk of harmful effects and that the risk is proportional to dose'. The chief of radiotherapy at the Cancer Institute in New York, Dr Robert Barish, has suggested that frequent fliers should be classified as 'occupationally exposed radiation workers'.

At around 40,000 ft the cosmic-ray impact is 100 times stronger than it is at sea level. In theory it is passengers on supersonic aircraft like Concorde who should be most worried, as the extra height that the aircraft flies at means that they receive around double the dosage experienced on a normal flight, but in practice the fact that Concorde travels at around twice the speed of any other airliner cuts the travelling time in half and thus equals out the effect. The problem is that, although the exposure to radiation on a single flight is not normally huge, the effect of exposure to radiation is cumulative, so that a frequent flier could easily accumulate an amount of exposure that constitutes a real risk.

The impact of absorbed radiation is measured in sieverts, but these are impractically large units, so human exposure is notched up in millisieverts (mSv) – thousandths of a sievert. The NRPB recommends that the maximum a member of the public should be exposed to from a single new source is 0.3 mSv per year. This is equivalent to an annual risk of 1 in 100,000 of contracting fatal cancer. In total, above the background level of radiation, the NRPB says the public should be limited to 1 mSv per year. For workers in special industries looser limits apply. The legal limit is 50 mSv per year, but the NRPB suggests a cap at 20 mSv per year – the equivalent of an annual risk of 1 in 1,000 of contracting fatal cancer. It also recommends that anyone receiving over 15 mSv per year should be put under close observation.

On Concorde, the cosmic-radiation level (which stays fairly constant, though all radiation is stronger when under the thinner atmospheric protection of polar flights) is around 0.01 mSv per hour. For an ordinary aircraft it is about half this. On top, however, has to be added the effect of the sun, which varies wildly. At the height of a solar storm (see page 140), the impact can be 1 mSv per hour or greater. Under times of peak solar activity this makes it easy for a frequent flier to exceed the recommended limits.

Quick Tip: **Special Hazards**

Radiation is known to be particularly dangerous to foetuses in the stages of organ development during the first three months of pregnancy. Pregnant women are advised to minimize the amount of time spent in the air (or in other increased-radiation environments) during this period.

The radiation workers

It may seem unfair that workers in some industries should be subject to a higher exposure limit, but the idea is that they are allowed this degree of exposure only if they are routinely monitored for the impact of radiation. Workers in this category include aircrew – in fact their exposure level is typically twice as much as the average worker in the nuclear industry. The casual flier is, of course, not monitored in this way.

Recent studies show that the dangers of radiation for frequent fliers are more than theoretical. A US survey of 6,000 flight attendants showed 30 per cent more incidence of breast cancer in the female staff than in the ordinary population. Skin cancer in male attendants was twice as high as normal. While it is always difficult to attribute a cause in a study like this – the increase in skin cancer may be because flight attendants spend more time on stopovers in exotic locations than the general public – it does seem likely that a contributory factor was the extra radiation exposure suffered by crew.

While even the most frequent business fliers will not clock up as many miles as the typical crew member, there is no doubt that they too are at an increased radiation risk.

In the background

Air travel is not the only context in which the ordinary member of the public is exposed to radiation. An average UK background exposure is 2.5 mSv per year, but the natural radiation levels in areas with heavy concentrations of granite (such as Cornwall and Edinburgh) are significantly higher than this. The typical annual dose in Cornwall is around 7.8 mSv – more than three times the level in London. In fact the UK's average is relatively low – France, for example, averages about 4 mSv, while Finland averages over 7 mSv.

The highest known level of background radiation affecting a substantial population is in Kerala and Madras states in India, with annual averages of over 30 mSv per year. Still higher levels occur in thinly populated areas in Brazil, Iran and Sudan, with average exposures up to 38 mSv per year. Four places are known in India and Europe where natural background radiation gives dose rates of more than 50 mSv per year. However, in the areas of high concentration of the most dangerous natural source – radon – bad ventilation can result in levels of 100 mSv per year. Areas with such natural dangers are given assistance (for instance in improving the ventilation of housing), but at more normal background levels we don't worry too much, so why should we bother about radiation in the aircraft cabin?

We probably should give more consideration to the impact of these natural sources, but the reason why we need to worry about aircraft exposure *as well* is the cumulative nature of the problem. Repeated exposure means that the risk is growing and growing. A frequent flier with around ten hours a week in the air can add around 4 mSv per year to his or her exposure. This will push some people into a higher-risk category. There are no certainties here – there isn't a specific safe limit, but there is no doubt that it is sensible to keep your radiation dosage to a minimum. If frequent fliers happen to live in areas of high background radiation as well, the exposure is increased again. Taking a sensible approach to radiation exposure is not scaremongering: it is as much a part of preventive medicine as taking enough exercise and eating a sensible diet.

If you are trying to cut down your background dosage, apart from moving away from natural high-dose areas, there is one rather surprising other action you can take. Shellfish concentrate natural radioactive materials, so that people who consume large quantities of shellfish will add as much as 0.5 mSv per year to their exposure. Avoiding shellfish will reduce your exposure to radiation by the equivalent of about ten transatlantic flights.

Escaping and monitoring

To get a complete picture of your radiation exposure, it is essential to start with some knowledge of the background exposure where you live. More information can be obtained from the NRPB in the UK (0800 614529; see page 329 for its web site) and from equivalent agencies in other countries. (If in doubt, contact your government health department.)

On top of this, you should be able to work out your rough exposure on the basis of 0.005 mSv per hour of flying (so a seven-hour flight would add 0.035 mSv to your annual exposure). Check the result against the recommended limits above.

→ Fast Track:
Flying Hours and Exposure

This graph gives a quick view of the link between flying hours and radiation exposure.

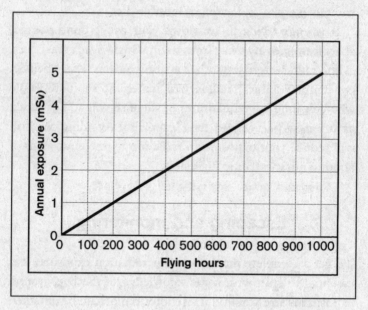

Bear in mind also that there is more exposure from the sun at times of peak solar activity. (At the time of writing we are just past a peak.) Because there is no consistency in the impact of solar radiation – it can be anything from negligible to a massive 1 mSv per hour – it isn't possible to add its effects into your calculation. All you can do is try to avoid solar storms and to reduce your flying hours during high-activity solar years. See below for more information on minimizing the chances of exposure to a solar storm.

→ Fast Track:
Check Your Radiation Exposure

Use this table to get a quick view of your exposure. Anything over 1mSv per year and you may want to look into monitoring your exposure.

Flights	Total exposure (mSv)
1 return trip from London to New York	0.07
1 return trip from London to Sydney	0.23
Monthly return trip from London to New York	0.89
Monthly return trip from London to Sydney	2.72
Weekly return trip from London to New York	3.77
Weekly return trip from London to Sydney	12.63
100 annual flying hours	0.5
500 annual flying hours	2.5
1,000 annual flying hours	5

If you have concerns about your exposure to radiation, you can get a small device that will monitor your cumulative levels through the year. The NRPB can provide and check these, as can a range of hospitals and specialists. In the UK, a full list of sources can be obtained from the Health and Safety Executive (08701 545500, see page 328 for its website). In other countries, contact the equivalent agency or your government health department.

Solar-weather watch

As the sun's output can, at its strongest, be by far the most significant source of radiation when flying, it helps to understand why the sun's radiation levels vary and how we can predict when it will have most impact. The surface of the sun is not an even, smooth sphere. Instead it is distorted by great storms that throw out masses of radioactive material into space, and emit waves of deadly radiation. These storms take place on an eleven-year cycle that last peaked in 2000.

The amount of radiation emitted at the peak of the cycle can be 100 times as high as in the troughs. Simply put, when we are in the peak of a cycle we are much more likely to be hit by a solar storm. Extreme storms can put radio stations out of operation. The earth is bombarded with much more radiation than normal. Mostly this is filtered out by the air, but the flier is exposed to more – around twice as much for each 2,000 m in height.

Like any forecasts, solar-weather forecasts rely on prob-

→ Fast Track:
The Solar Cycle

This graph gives an indication of the relative strength of the
sun's radiation through its eleven-year cycle.

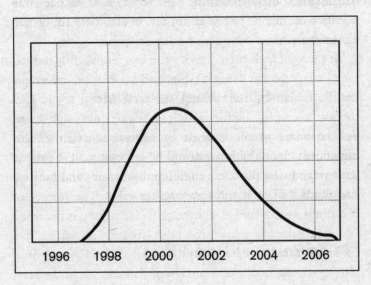

1996   1998   2000   2002   2004   2006

abilities, so there are no certainties. But if you already have
a high radiation exposure it would be worth considering
rescheduling a flight when a major flare is likely. You would
also be very sensible to look to reducing your flying hours
around peaks – between 1999 and 2003 (roughly), again in
2010 to 2014, and so on.

You can get up-to-date forecasts of solar weather and
the likelihood of solar flares at the Space Weather Bureau.
There is a lot of information on the Bureau's web site (see

page 329). (This is sometimes overloaded with jargon, but look out for the section labelled something like 'Space weather NOAA forecasts'.) You can also get direct information from the NOAA (the US National Oceanic and Atmospheric Agency – see page 329). Unless there is a warning of a major peak, the best advice is to reduce your number of flights per year in the higher periods of the eleven-year cycle.

At times of high solar activity you can also slightly reduce your exposure by flying at night. This has no effect on cosmic radiation, but will put the earth between you and the sun's output. Unfortunately, however, although there will be some small decrease in exposure, much of the impact of solar radiation will still be felt even on the earth's dark side, as the planet is engulfed in a jet of particles that surrounds it like a liquid surrounding a ball.

✈ *Summary:* **Bad Vibes**

- There is a real risk from the radiation exposure on aircraft.

- We are all exposed to background radiation – it is useful to know this background level to put your airline exposure in context.

- If you are trying to cut down on radiation exposure, cut shellfish out of your diet.

- Around 200 flying hours a year will bring you up to

the maximum radiation exposure recommended by the National Radiological Protection Board.

- Anyone undergoing more exposure to radioactivity should consider regular checks.

- Solar weather has a major effect on radiation. Avoid peaks, and reduce flying hours in heavy parts of the solar cycle.

8 Defeating the Lag

Until the early aviators began to make long journeys – such as Charles Lindbergh's thirty-three-hour crossing from New York to Paris in 1927, or Wiley Post's eight-day trip around the world in 1931 – the impact of different time zones on the human body had not really been considered. Before then, the lengthy crossing of oceans by ship had allowed time for the body to settle into new rhythms. With the introduction of the jet airliner in the 1950s it became possible to plunge into totally different time zones in a matter of hours. Jet lag was born.

Is there any such thing?

At the heart of the difficulty in getting a handle on jet lag is the fact that it is not a medical condition. Just as most of us are suspicious of miraculous mixtures of vitamins that are supposed to give us the energy we lack (when we know that what we really need is a few nights of good sleep and a healthy diet), we should treat any miracle cure for jet lag with caution. Jet lag can no more be 'cured' than being tired can. But, as with ordinary tiredness, we can either fool the body into thinking that the exhaustion does not exist or we can minimize its impact or even prevent it entirely by recognizing its true nature.

The primary component of jet lag is fatigue. The traveller is subject not only to the exacerbated weariness caused by reduced air pressure in the cabin, but also to the tiredness and disorientation of a shift worker who has to switch sleeping patterns away from the norm. In fact, in an article on jet lag in December 1984 in *Aviation, Space and Environmental Medicine*, a group of NASA scientists highlight just how many similarities there are between the symptoms of jet lag and of shift working. While it seems true that jet lag is made worse by dehydration, and perhaps by reduced cabin air pressure, we are not dealing with something inherently connected with travelling to far-off places, nor do we have to cope with a disease.

Yet this simple fact should not be allowed to diminish the potential difficulties caused by jet lag. If you are travelling on business, you do not want to be performing under par at your destination. A classic example of the danger of jet lag comes from the late John Foster Dulles, one-time Secretary of State of the USA. Dulles admitted that he had precipitated the Suez Crisis by making a decision to cancel a loan to Egypt for the Aswan Dam immediately after his return to Washington from the Middle East. He did not allow himself time to recover from jet lag, and considered this to be the primary cause of his mistake.

Coping with the lag

Unfortunately, few of us can simply wait for the symptoms of jet lag to go away. It takes around a day to overcome each hour of time zone crossed – that's getting on for a week for a transatlantic flight alone. The effect seems slightly less pronounced when flying in a westerly direction. As some of our natural body cycles operate on a longer period than the twenty-four hours of a day, adding to the day by catching up with the sun seems to be less traumatic. But, realistically, this knowledge is not much use if you want to travel to the East. Some suggest wearing dark glasses when flying in this direction, but there is little evidence that this helps.

The best proven method to counter the effects of jet lag is to control food and water intake and to take a sensible approach to sleep. The procedure begins before you get on board. Get as much sleep as you can before flying. Don't eat heavily or drink to excess for twenty-four hours before your flight. What you do eat on that day before is up to you, but keep it to food that you would think of as bland and safe. You might love spicy curries, but a vindaloo is not a good idea the night before a long-haul flight.

Action on board

On the plane, your first action should be to set your watch to your destination time and operate from that immediately, rather than working to any schedule that the cabin crew try to operate. A one-time courier for the British Foreign Office emphasizes the importance of this:

> As soon as you get on the aircraft, put your watch to the destination time and arrange your sleep pattern to fit in with the destination. In other words, if you are arriving in the morning, make sure that you have had about six hours' sleep before you land. If you are arriving in the evening, make sure that you have been awake for about eight hours beforehand. For arrival time in between this, adjust accordingly. Sounds like a cooking recipe, doesn't it?
>
> When you get to your destination, get into the local time immediately and, whatever you do, don't have a lie-in – it will waste all the preparation. This method can mean that you don't take full advantage of the in-flight catering. No hardship. If you are in first or club [business class] they normally rustle up something to your convenience anyway.

There is one exception to this approach. If you are diabetic, it may be wiser to stick on your home time zone for meals during your whole stay away. (This can obviously be difficult in practice.) Get appropriate medical advice before travelling.

As the courier suggests, it is best to sleep when it makes sense in terms of your destination time zone. If you start operating on the new time as soon as possible, your body will get used to the change much quicker – and you won't suffer from time shock when you step off the plane and discover that there is bright sunlight when you thought it was two in the morning.

Quick Tip: Belt Out

If you use a blanket when you sleep on the plane, it's a good idea to fasten your seat belt loosely outside the blanket rather than under it. That way, if there's turbulence, the crew won't need to disturb you to check that you are safely strapped in.

It might seem tempting to try to control your sleep pattern with sleeping pills. Perhaps you feel that this will help you to get a good sleep on the plane itself, despite the uncomfortable seat and all the distractions. Perhaps you might see it as a way to reschedule your sleeping after landing. In practice this has proved an ineffective solution. During flight it's not a good idea to be in a drugged sleep. At least when you are dozing you can move regularly to minimize the impact of the seat on your legs. And there is always the very small possibility of an emergency, in which case you would want to be able to wake fully without effort. At your destination, forcing sleep with pills slows down your recovery from jet lag rather than enhancing it. All the evidence is that sleeping pills are an ineffective way to overcome jet lag.

Keep your food consumption on the plane down to a minimum. Drink as much water as you can during flight (and remember to drink extra before you go to sleep). It is better to stick to still water even if you enjoy the carbonated version more, as the gas build-up in the gut is made worse by the low cabin pressure. Aircraft carry a limited supply of bottled water, so it is worth taking your own bottle in your cabin bag, particularly if you are travelling economy. I have found recently that the cabin crew at the expensive end of the cabin have caught on to the idea of regular water input, and will regularly top up a glass with bottled water for business- and first-class passengers throughout a flight. Just make sure you don't let them take your glass away, and they will usually get the hint.

Unfortunately, depending on the airline's bottled water does involve an element of trust. In a 1997 *Wall Street Journal* article, United Airlines was accused of filling water bottles from the tap for its business customers. Drinking on-board tap water is not a great idea, as it is untreated and there is no guarantee it won't be full of bugs. Studies have found that around 25 per cent of aircraft have tainted tap water, probably because the tanks aren't cleaned often enough and are filled rather casually by engineers on the tarmac. If you have any concerns, stick to your own bottled water.

Space invaders

Sleeping and aircraft seats rarely go well together, and there are issues of increased risk from deep-vein thrombosis (see page 91), but in principle sleeping is a good way to spend some of the flight time, provided you match your sleeping hours to the time at your destination.

Quick Tip: **Lavender Time**

An aromatherapy classic that has proved more reliable than most is the use of lavender oil to relax and aid sleep. A tiny phial of lavender will last a whole trip – put a few drops on an upper garment or pillow on the plane to improve the chances of sleep. It's also a benefit in hotel bedrooms. Several top airlines now provide lavender oil in their first-class washbags. If lavender helps you drift off at the right time it will also help counter jet lag.

These days, airlines use sophisticated inventory-management systems to try to maximize the number of paying bodies that are occupying their seats, but there will still be some empty seats on most flights. These provide an opportunity for the luxury of space if attacked in the right way. What's more, you may not have managed to get allocated a seat in your favourite position, yet one might be free on the flight, perhaps because a passenger didn't show up.

Although your boarding pass will specify a seat, after take-off you have no obligation to stay in that seat if another is vacant. The cabin crew often try to ensure that you stay in your allocated seat until then, as the balance of the aircraft will have been calculated on the assumption that that is where you will be. This is a less critical problem on landing, when the aircraft will be significantly less heavy due to all the fuel that has been burned up – hence the crew's short-term interest.

It may be that you win the lottery and already have two vacant seats next to you. If so, go for the middle seat, fasten your belt loosely, and lift up the arms on either side to

---

Quick Tip: **Pillow Talk**

Getting to sleep on an aircraft is inevitably a battle. A pillow will usually help. If you aren't given one, ask the cabin crew – they may be able to provide one. Passengers with window seats have one advantage over the others – they have the wall of the aircraft to prop them up (although the bigger seats in business and first class often have 'wings' to support the head).

Some passengers swear by inflatable neck pillows that sit on the shoulders and are supposed to help you rest in almost any position. I find them constricting, but they're worth a try. The same goes for eyeshades. Many regular travellers think they are wonderful, but I feel uncomfortable and disoriented when wearing them.

The temperature on board an aircraft varies considerably. It is useful to have several layers of clothes, so you can put layers on and take them off to get a suitable temperature for sitting and for sleeping. A blanket almost always comes in useful – ask the cabin crew if you haven't been provided with one.

make a not exactly comfortable but practical bed. (Apart from cheapness, this is about the only advantage of travelling economy class – the fancy seats in business and first are too solid to have arms that you can lift up.) Alternatively, look out for empty blocks of seats where you can stretch out – often more likely in the wider mid-section of a large jet. You need to be assertive, claiming the seats as your right, and quick or others will get there first. But bear in mind that there is a limit to realistic pushiness. If someone else is already sitting next to the vacant seat it would be bad manners to claim it as your own.

One reason why you might want to stay in your original seat even if you spot a luxurious gap is that the crew are given a sheet of paper that identifies who is sitting where, and any special requirements that the passengers might have. If you have ordered a special meal, or have special medical requirements like supplementary oxygen, it makes things simpler if you stick with your allocated seat.

Using the break

If you have a transit stop, you are being given an opportunity to minimize the impact of jet lag (and of deep-vein thrombosis). Make use of the chance to be out of the confines of the aircraft, to walk around and get as much exercise as you can.

A transit stop is also an opportunity to work on your dehydration. Keep up the water intake while on the ground. Get exposure to natural light if you can. But don't think that your meal regimen is over – treat eating in a transit stop as you would eating on the plane.

Back on the ground

On reaching your destination, some experts suggest that it is OK to have a short nap, but my experience is that any amount of sleep helps disturb your rhythms and you wake up feeling worse than you did before. It's a struggle, but you should stick with the local time. Get some exercise as soon as you arrive. An ideal way to do this is to take a walk around.

Typically you will have been shuttled to a hotel by taxi or by bus. You will have no context for where you are. Psychologically, taking a walk around your location will help you overcome the feeling of strangeness and displacement that aggravates jet lag. It also gets you out of the air-conditioned environment, and perhaps most of all gives you exposure to natural light, which seems to be one of the best ways to encourage your body cycles to synchronize with a new environment.

If you have forced yourself to keep awake and have taken some exercise, the chances are that by the time you get to bedtime at your destination you will be tired. It may be that you will wake up briefly in the night, but most people who have tried the sensible approach to overcoming jet lag find that they can get back to sleep without a problem. If you experience difficulty getting that sleepy feeling, don't reach for the sleeping tablets (see above) –

try a soak in a warm bath and a suitably boring book as bedtime reading.

Eat at normal (local) times. One advantage of minimizing food intake on the aircraft is that you will really be ready for your meal when you land, making it easier to synchronize with local eating times. It is often suggested that the on-board food is best avoided altogether, perhaps because activating the digestion takes over some of the body's oxygen intake and so increases the impact of the low oxygen levels. This wouldn't have an input on sleep patterns, but could result in feeling mildly unwell or irritable after the flight.

I can't say that I have found this to be the case. Provided you are sensible, it is quite possible to eat on board and still avoid jet lag. It can be particularly difficult to say no to food, much more so than to offers of alcohol or coffee – it is hard to avoid the feeling that you are abusing someone's hospitality. And sometimes, even though you know it is convenience food, the offerings on the trolley can smell quite good.

The best approach is to be selective. Only eat if you feel hungry, not just for the sake of it. Try to go for food that's high in carbohydrates, as these seem to be the most effective food at high altitudes on the evidence of mountain climbers. Go for bread and cereals at breakfast time, and concentrate on potatoes, pasta or rice in a hot meal. Fruit that's high in water and not too acidic – such as melon and watermelon – is pretty good too. Don't eat everything you're given just because it's there.

→ Fast Track:
Beating Jet Lag

• Eat light meals of bland food on the day before departure.

• Set your time to the destination as soon as you board the aircraft (except diabetics – see page 147).

• Keep food consumption on board down to a minimum. Stick to high-carbohydrate snacks.

• Drink at least a glass of bottled water an hour.

• Sleep and eat on board in keeping with your destination time.

• On arrival, get out into natural light and exercise.

• Don't go to sleep at your destination until the normal time for that location.

Popping the pills

The alternative to dealing with jet lag properly is to hide its effects, just as consuming coffee and other stimulants may be able temporarily to mitigate the effects of normal tiredness. Recently there have been a number of studies into the level of benefit provided by the anti-jet-lag drug melatonin. This pineal hormone is said to fool the brain into ignoring the impact of changing time zones. Research at the University of Heidelberg has shown that after a long flight there are changes in the body's levels of melatonin. There is a strong link between melatonin levels and ability to sleep. But there are real questions attached to the prescribing of melatonin as a 'cure' for jet lag. According to one of the UK's leading medical journals, the *Lancet*, in 1986, 'Its apparent usefulness in alleviating the effects of jet lag may be related to some ill-defined psychotropic activity [i.e. activity affecting one's mental state], but such effects may be undesirable, particularly if they modify daytime function . . . It also has endocrine [upsetting the hormonal balance in the body] effects . . . The effects cannot be dismissed lightly . . .'

If the drug works at all, it is necessary to stick to a rigid timing programme of doses around your flight time. Get the schedule wrong and the drug will make jet lag worse instead of improving your response. More worryingly, however, as with any hormonal treatment, there is considerable concern about possible side effects. When compared with a non-invasive approach like the one suggested above, the use of melatonin seems doubtful at best.

If you do want to try melatonin, it is available over the counter in US health shops, but requires a doctor's prescription in the UK. Be aware that to get any benefit from it you not only need to stick to the timing regime but also to take the drug under dim lighting conditions.

Alternative jet-lag cures

There is at least some evidence that melatonin has an effect, even if the possible side effects may be worse than the original problem. By contrast, some suggested jet-lag cures are based entirely on subjective supposition. There is a whole range of alternative therapies and exotic treatments available. Some involve a complex fast-and-feast diet process for days in advance. Others involve shining bright lights on the traveller to confuse his or her natural rhythms. Perhaps the only ones worth considering are mechanisms like aromatherapy and homoeopathy (see page 34) that can be seen as a complement to the simple sleep-and-water approach. Anything that helps you get off to sleep in a natural way should be beneficial.

Some exotic ideas have also been used to explain the less documented problem of north–south jet lag. Conventional jet lag arises on flights that involve crossing time zones, but what of long-distance flights that don't result in a change of time? If time shift were the sole cause of jet lag, there should be no effect produced by long-distance flights from north to south or from south to north. But there is.

This has led some writers on air travel to suppose the existence of bizarre influences. They point out that travellers from north to south or from south to north experience a shift in the earth's magnetic fields. They note that water (a major part of the body, after all) seems to act differently north and south of the Equator, as shown by the way that it runs down the plughole clockwise in the north and anticlockwise in the south. The conclusion is that being in a different hemisphere may have a direct effect on our bodily fluids.

Unfortunately, such fascinating ideas have little basis in scientific reality. The bathwater's direction of spin is supposed to be caused by the Coriolis force – an impressive-sounding concept, though nothing more than a side effect of the earth's rotation. In fact this force is very weak, and all the evidence is that the supposed difference in direction of water going down the plughole is imaginary – whether it runs clockwise or anticlockwise is much more likely to be determined by chaotic motion in the flow of the fluid: the influence of the Coriolis force is very slight. And, although there is some evidence that homing pigeons are influenced by magnetic fields, the earth's field is not strong and again is unlikely to have any impact on our well-being.

Instead of being baffled by pseudo-science, we just need to look back at what jet lag really is – disorientation similar to that of a shift worker, coupled with fatigue due to time change, the impact of dehydration, and exposure to low air pressure. All of these factors except for the time-based disorientation are still present in a long flight in a single time zone. There is no need for any mystical force to provide a weaker form of jet lag in north-to-south and south-to-north long-haul passengers. Nor is there a need for a different cure.

✈ *Summary*: Defeating the Lag

- Jet lag is not an illness: it is a combination of fatigue, dehydration, the effects of low pressure, and the disorientation felt by shift workers.

- Jet lag takes around a day to overcome fully for each hour of time zone crossed.

- The effect of jet lag is slightly less pronounced when flying west.

- Changing over to local time immediately on entering the plane, minimizing food intake, and only drinking water will help a lot.

- Don't sleep at the destination until the normal local time.

- Although melatonin has some useful effects, all the evidence is that the risk is not worth the benefits.

- Sleeping pills have entirely the wrong result for overcoming jet lag.

- Apart from the lack of time difference, the same causes produce north–south jet lag as generate the east–west effect.

9 Flight Stress, Fear of Flying and Air Rage

Flying is stressful. It's not surprising. You are trapped in a metal tube, thousands of feet up in the air, with no control and no way out. In a 1984 Swedish survey on the fear of flying, although only 25 per cent of people admitted to a general sense of apprehension when airborne, tension soared in twice that number during landing. For inexperienced fliers the figures are even worse, peaking at around three-quarters when experiencing turbulence. Even if you aren't actually scared of flying, the whole business of getting through an airport and on to a plane can generate plenty of pressure. Such stress is not just a factor in turning flight into an unpleasant experience – it increases the risk of medical problems, especially those related to the heart, the respiratory system and the nervous system. Furthermore, it can precipitate the syndrome known as air rage.

Fear is normal

Although they may not admit it, most people feel fear at some time during flight. This anxiety is not helped by the dismissive approach of some aviation 'experts'. It is all too common to hear comments like 'Most people are actually still frightened of flying. It's an irrational fear. They don't understand why aeroplanes stay up in the air.' Not only is this an incorrect analysis, it manages to be patronizing as well. The fear of flying is perfectly rational. We all feel some apprehension when in high places as a matter of self-preservation – and only an astronaut is ever going to get higher than the occupants of a plane. The very thought of being eleven kilometres above the ground is enough to give anyone a sense of dread.

What the so-called expert was identifying was not a lack of knowledge so much as an awareness of engineering fallibility. It has nothing to do with failing to understand the mechanics of flight and everything to do with understanding the mechanics of falling. The basis for fear is not ignorance of aerodynamics but the knowledge that a plane is a complex mechanism with thousands of parts designed by fallible humans, assembled by fallible humans, and maintained by fallible humans. Things can go wrong, and this is a perfectly legitimate source of fear.

But – and it's a big but – once the real object of fear is identified, something can be done about it. Because, in comparison with the risks we take every day, flying is not a bad bet. It's a natural human reaction for fear to increase when we hear about danger. In the two weeks after the United Airlines Flight 232 accident in 1989 (see page 232), sales for tickets on flights using the McDonnell Douglas DC-10 aircraft type that was involved in the crash decreased by 36 per cent. But such a reaction needs a rational counter argument. As is explored in more detail in Chapter 16, the chances of being killed in a crash on a particular flight are better than 8 million to 1 – not bad odds, comparable with those of being killed by a stroke of lightning.

But, although it's fine to appeal to logic in this way, the fact is that people's behaviour often fails to take account of statistical reality. The number of people who regularly go in for major lotteries with the expectation of winning, when the chances may be tens of millions to one, demonstrates this. And there is always the perfectly logical point put across by some of those who hate flying (famous people who have refused to fly at all included film director Stanley Kubrick, science-fiction author Isaac Asimov and Dutch footballer Dennis Bergkamp) that, whatever the level of risk, you are even less likely to be involved in a plane crash if you never get on a plane. Even so, when the reality of the statistics is combined with some on-the-day techniques it is usually possible to keep the fear of flying under control.

White-knuckle sound effects

For new fliers there are sights and particularly sounds that can trigger anxiety. Being aware of what to expect will help keep these worries in check. Just realizing that a plane's wings are supposed to flex, to move around gently in flight, can help. Similarly, the collection of bumps and bangs that always accompany flight can be made less fearsome if they are expected.

→ Fast Track: Noises Off

Air travel is accompanied by a range of noises that can be frankly unnerving for the inexperienced flier. Being aware of the source of the sounds that will accompany flight makes it easier to ignore them.

Stage of flight	Noise	What's happening?
On the stand	Grinding noise followed by loud bang from under the aircraft. The whole plane often shakes.	Baggage hatches are being shut.
Before moving	Vibration, engine noise	When the engines first start up they can seem surprisingly noisy.
While taxiing	Creaks and rattles	It can be something of a shock that the plane sounds like a rusty old spring as it creaks over the bumps in the taxiway – but this is perfectly normal.
Nearing the runway	A bell-like alarm briefly sounds	Nothing has gone wrong: this is just the captain giving a last warning of take-off to the cabin crew.
Turning on to the runway	Sudden roar of engine noise	If the runway is clear ahead, the captain will often opt for a 'running start', opening the throttles wide as soon as the plane is pointed down the runway. This is entirely safe.

During take-off	Significant vibration; rattles from the galley and bumps from the tyres	Runways are always pretty bumpy. Take-off will involve vibration, and particularly rattles from loose metal like the cooking trays in the galley.
Shortly after take-off	Engine noises quietens as if the plane is losing power	The pilot is obliged to reduce thrust as soon as possible after take-off, to cut down noise for those who live near the airport. It is normal procedure.
Shortly after take-off	Whine accompanied by 'grinding' vibration followed by one or more thumps	Once the pilot is sure he isn't going to have to go straight back and land, the landing gear is lifted into the aircraft body to make it more streamlined.
During cruising	Sudden increase of engine noise	Occasionally during cruising the flight crew will be asked by air traffic control to change altitude, as airspace is split into 'corridors' that have depth as well as width. Changing height will result in unexpected changes in engine noise.
Shortly before landing	Engine noise drops off to almost nothing	After a long flight it will seem as if the engines have cut out as the noise dies back. The plane has to slow down and lose height to land – this is all that is happening.
Shortly before landing	Whining accompanied by 'grinding' vibration from both wings and below aircraft	As well as the landing gear opening out, the flight crew will extend the flaps on the wing, enabling the aircraft to fly at a lower speed for landing. The hydraulic motors produce this noise.

Just before landing (very occasionally)	Engines begin to produce a loud roar; plane starts to pull away from the ground	Very occasionally the plane's landing will be aborted. Usually this is because a plane in front has not cleared the runway. This is a simple procedure for the flight crew, who will simply bring the plane around for another landing.
On the runway	A thump, followed by a very loud roar from the engines	As the plane hits the runway there is often a thump – but the tyres are designed to take this. Then the pilot puts the engines into reverse to brake the aircraft, hence the loud roar.

In part the nervousness produced by the sounds and movements of the plane is a direct result of relying on technology to keep you up in the air. It is also true, though, that the view from a typical aircraft seat gives a misleading impression of your surroundings, and this itself can be unnerving. Windows in aircraft involve a compromise between visibility and safety. To make sure that they can survive the strains of pressurization, they are thick and small. Your view is very restricted. At the time of writing it is not possible for passengers to get access to the flight deck, but should it become feasible, ask for a visit. It is worth taking this action, because the pilots' view is so much better. The glass is clear. You can see around, above, below. Because there isn't such a restrictive field of vision, there is a much greater feeling of stability, of safety. You will probably also be reassured by the calm inaction on the flight deck. During cruising, a modern airliner pretty well flies itself. The crew are relaxed, though ready to deal with any eventuality. It *feels* safe.

A bouncy ride

After take-off and landing, the most stressful time is when the aircraft undergoes turbulence. Even mild turbulence can seem frightening. The aircraft begins to buck and shake. It is as if you are rattling along a very bumpy road – but you know that you are perhaps ten kilometres up in the air. Some turbulence can be even more dramatic, throwing the plane at a sudden angle, or dropping it hundreds of feet like a stone. For any flier, even the most experienced, this can be a terrifying time.

It would be foolish to say that turbulence is harmless. It has killed people in the past. But the first reassurance has to be that the chances of it causing the plane to crash are almost zero. Among all the jet-airliner fatalities caused by turbulence between 1980 and 1997 (the statistics exclude the old Soviet Union countries, where accurate data is hard to come by), only one involved a plane – a small Fokker F28 City Hopper – actually crashing as a result of the turbulence. The height at which jets fly gives a lot of leeway to recover from the most severe turbulence.

In fact the danger from turbulence results from being thrown around within the aircraft cabin. In the five events resulting in deaths other than the Fokker crash between 1980 and 1997, either one or two passengers were killed –

> ## *Quick Tip:* Heads Up
>
> *If you have a seat that is directly under an overhead locker, be very wary whenever anyone goes to open it. No doubt you have been careful and not put anything heavy up there, but you can't guarantee the thoughtfulness of your fellow passengers. After the contents of the locker have been thoroughly shaken up – by bouncing down the runway, steep climbs, and the sudden lurches of turbulence – it is quite possible that something may be propped against the locker door, ready to drop on your head as it is opened.*
>
>   *This is not a trivial consideration. People have been killed by heavy objects (briefcases, for example) plunging from a locker and breaking their necks. If someone heads for the locker, keep an eye on what they are doing, and keep your head out of the way.*

generally because they were not strapped into their seat. (Occasionally injury is caused by flying objects, particularly if one or more overhead lockers burst open.) The message is simple: keep your seat belt fastened at all times (even when the 'Fasten seat belts' sign isn't lit) and you will immediately remove the majority of the risk from turbulence.

The flight crew will give you warning if possible, but their weather radar only spots certain kinds of turbulence. The sudden impact of clear-air turbulence, for example, comes entirely (and literally) out of the blue.

Staying strapped in is great advice in theory, but at times you need to get up, if only to go to the toilet. If the 'Fasten seat belts' signs are on I would recommend holding on for a few minutes – often a burst of turbulence lasts only a short time. There is no guarantee that there won't still be turbulence after the sign goes off, but at least you can reduce your chances of being thrown about.

The art of distraction

The easiest method of dealing with the fear of flying is to employ distraction. This is the approach that the airlines take all the time. From the moment you reach your seat until you get off the plane there will be various attempts to distract you from your seemingly fragile environment.

The airline's two main means of distraction are the in-flight entertainment and food and drink. Unfortunately (see page 119) the airline's insistence on pouring drinks down you (especially alcoholic drinks) and its rigid schedule of meals are particularly bad for other aspects of surviving the flight. It is best to make use of your own distractions to supplement the in-flight entertainment.

It is hard to beat reading as a way of taking yourself away from your surroundings. I have seen it suggested that magazines make better in-flight reading than books, because you can throw them away at the end of the flight. But magazines don't offer the same level of immersion that books do, especially a good page-turner that keeps you glued to the plot. A better tactic is to use paperbacks that you don't mind discarding after use.

Work too can act as a distraction, though, as we have seen (page 104), the reduced level of oxygen on the aircraft can mean that it is difficult to concentrate, making it all too easy to end up reading the same phrase over and over again. The main thing is that you should be aware of the need for distraction and take action to keep your mind occupied.

I find the most difficult time can be when lying awake while attempting to get off to sleep. It is all too easy to start thinking about how precarious your position is, particularly if a bout of turbulence brews up at this point. In these circumstances the best technique seems to be consciously to force yourself to think of something else, squashing any tendency to drift back to your location above the clouds.

Basic relaxation

Fear itself is not necessarily the worst aspect of the natural reaction to flying. Fear causes stress, and this negative stress has a bad effect on your health, particularly if you are at risk of stress-influenced medical conditions like heart problems. The whole experience of flying is inherently stressful, making stress control an important part of the armoury of any flier. Where the stressor is fear, there are two tactics that can be used: removing the fear (perhaps by distraction) and countering the impact of stress. Perhaps the easiest way to do this is through relaxation.

Quick Tip: Simple Breathing

A simple breathing exercise will reduce stress almost instantly and can be undertaken practically anywhere. First find your diaphragmatic breathing. Take a deep breath and hold it for a second. Your chest will rise. Now try to keep your chest in the 'up position' while breathing in and out. You should feel a tensing and relaxing around the stomach area. Rest a hand gently on your stomach to feel it in action. You are breathing with your diaphragm – a much more controlled, relaxing process than chest breathing.

Now get as comfortable as you can. Close your eyes if possible. Begin to breathe regularly. Count up to five (in your head!) as you breathe in through your nose. Hold it for a second, then breathe out through your mouth, again counting to five. Rest a hand on your stomach. Don't consciously force your ribcage to stay up now, but concentrate on movement of the diaphragm. Your stomach should gently rise as you breathe in and fall as you breathe out. Keep going for a couple of minutes before gradually opening your eyes.

Any exercises suggested to help reduce the impact of deep-vein thrombosis (see page 94, for example) are also likely to be useful for dealing with stress.

The whole stress package

In all there are four ways to counter stress. The first is to remove the stressor. In this case the answer would be not to fly. That might not be an option that is available to you, but it is something to consider where there are alternatives. If you hate flying and need to get from London to Paris, use Eurostar instead. If flying is stressful for you, use it when you must (for example on a business trip), but consider taking a holiday somewhere that doesn't require you to take to the air. After all, unless you indulge in extreme sports, the purpose of a holiday is to reduce your stress levels, not make them worse.

If you can't remove the source of stress entirely, there are three options to counter the effects of the stress, working on the physical, emotional and spiritual levels.

Because stress is a physiological response to the stressor, it is subject to physical control. At the extreme this can mean resorting to drugs, but it can also be achieved by giving the body the natural defences it needs to cope well with the impact of stress. Human beings have never before had such a sedentary life. Much work is now chair-bound, whether you are sitting in front of a computer screen or driving a car. The TV ensures that our entertainment is often low-energy too. We don't walk as much as we used to. Recent reports have shown that women, who traditionally had less of a problem with diseases caused by insufficient exercise, have now caught up with men. A major factor in being able to deal with stress is improving your physical condition. Often this involves basics like better sleep, better eating and more exercise.

There are also physical controls that go beyond basic health improvements. Many find massage particularly effective (some airlines, like Virgin, offer in-flight massage in business class). The benefits of aromatherapy may not be entirely proven, but many people feel it does work for them, and, bearing in mind the nature of stress, the perception of benefit is enough to make it worth trying.

Although we tend to think of stress as very much an internal thing, we shouldn't ignore these physical aids. There's a limit to how much physical action can be taken to counter stress during a flight, but taking more physical care in the weeks leading up to travel really can have an impact. However, a lot more can be done to help with stress coming not from the body, but from the mind.

The stress inside

Much of our response to stress depends on our emotional state and self-image. If we are depressed and unhappy, stress will have a disproportionately large impact. We've all been in the position of snapping at someone for a very minor offence when we are already feeling miserable. Help with your emotional state can make all the difference to how you cope with stress. Similarly, self-confidence and feeling in control of your life are immensely valuable when it comes to fending off negative stress. Something as apparently flimsy as attitude and self-esteem has a very big impact.

Taking the time to examine the areas where you feel out of control is an excellent starting point in taking emotional control of stress. Look for opportunities to do things *your* way, rather than *their* way. Work on your self-image, giving yourself a conscious pat on the back each time you achieve something (and, with a little thought, we can all identify achievements every day). Taking emotional control isn't a quick fix – it may involve major changes to how you live your life – but it is one of the best ways to keep stress in its place. If you feel in need of assistance with emotional

---

Quick Tip: **Find your Anchors**

Modern life is fast-paced, full of change and stress. Air travel magnifies this. In themselves, change and pace are not bad things. Even stress, in controlled amounts, is not bad – it is the source of all challenge, it is what gives life zest. The important thing is to have a balance.

Stress gets out of control when we don't make enough of our anchors, the still points in our world of change. Consciously identify your anchors. They might be major ones like your family, your profession or your religion. They might include rituals like a glass of red wine in the evening or following a football team. Be clear what your personal anchors are, and make sure that they occupy the front of your mind when you are under stress. Your anchors will help put the causes of stress into perspective.

control, look out a stress-management book, such as my own *Instant Stress Management* (Kogan Page).

Equally important is the potential of having spiritual barriers to help resist and overcome stress. There's a dichotomy in our world. We have never been more rational, scientific and analytical. Yet everyone will at some time feel a yearning for something more, something beyond the everyday. This need for something more has led to a huge interest in everything from New Age philosophy to established religions.

The specific approach taken isn't really of concern here. The important consideration is the power of having a spiritual dimension to your life in helping control stress. Many religions emphasize prayer or meditation as a means of building spiritual calm, which has the practical effect of reducing the impact of stress. An appropriate prayer or mantra has helped many fearful fliers to cope. In fact, properly used, such spiritual tools can be the most effective stress-relievers. Accepting a spiritual dimension to your life can also help overcome difficulties with the 'big issues' that are rarely thought about or discussed in ordinary life and so remain a nagging worry on the threshold of consciousness. Death is inevitably one of these big issues and lies behind the fear of flying. Don't dismiss the spiritual content of your stress-relief package.

Getting it taped

An option that falls between distraction and stress relief is to use a relaxation tape to help overcome the tension of fear and to dismiss thoughts of possible problems. There are many specially produced tapes designed to aid relaxation, some involving elements of subliminal suggestion (though I can't vouch for the value of this).

I personally find the content of most relaxation tapes musically distressing, and would recommend trying a few alternatives that could be equally effective. I particularly value pre-classical church music, featuring either the soothing, chanting rhythms of plainsong or the more sophisticated intertwining of Tudor and Elizabethan (Renaissance) masterpieces. Allegri's *Miserere* is probably the best-known piece in this style, though almost anything by composers like Byrd, Gibbons, Palestrina, Sheppard, Tallis, Taverner and Tye is equally effective.

Much classical music or modern serious music is also very soothing if you keep away from vigorous or blaring orchestrations. Look for calm, reflective pieces – a lot of the earlier twentieth-century English composers like Delius and Elgar wrote plenty of works along these lines. There is also a lot of relaxation value in the surging, repetitive themes of modern composers like Michael Nyman (responsible for the score of the film *The Piano*), John Tavener and TV composer Barrington Pheloung (who wrote the music for the *Inspector Morse* series).

A final option is to look at folk music and downbeat jazz.

In a recent test, John Denver's music was found to be among the most relaxing in existence. You might not like it, but it's easy to see how it can help the listener to switch off.

→ Fast Track:
  Stress and Fear

- Understand the noises a plane makes.

- Be aware of the lack of danger (if strapped in) from turbulence.

- Distract yourself with entertainment and appropriate work.

- Use simple relaxation exercises.

- Find your personal anchors.

- Look at physical, emotional and spiritual de-stressors.

- Try relaxation tapes.

The impossible fear

For some people, flying is more than a simple cause of stress – it is the subject of a phobia. Around 10 per cent of the population won't go near a plane. Some don't discover just how bad their fear is until they are queuing up at the gate, only to find that they are unable to get on board. The same Swedish study that discovered this fact pointed out that 38 per cent of people said they had a close friend or relative who refused to fly. The authors of the study inferred that the percentage who wouldn't fly was higher than was admitted, because people were referring to themselves indirectly. In fact, though, it's hardly surprising that many of us have friends and relations who won't fly. There's only one individual to choose from when answering a question about one's own attitudes, but everyone has a range of friends and relations, probably making the observation in the Swedish study statistically irrelevant.

For some people it is enough to tackle fear of flying with the same relaxation or distraction techniques that work for everyday fear. For others the phobia may never be conquered. However, there are courses for fearful fliers that can help. British Airways supports the course run by Aviatours (01252 793250), which includes a short flight of approximately one-hour duration conducted by an experienced British Airways training captain, following preparation by a clinical psychologist. Similar courses are offered in the UK by Britannia Airways (01582 424155) and Virgin Atlantic (01293 448440). In other countries, ring the customer-services department of a major airline for suggestions.

Whether you just feel a twinge of anxiety or succumb to out-and-out terror, something to remember is that fear of flying *is* a perfectly natural fear. You are not being cowardly. Instead you are reacting in a way that is normal for a human being. As with other natural human reactions, you can probably use your will to overcome the fear, but it is natural. And it can happen to anyone, whether first-time fliers or those with great experience. Pilots who have flown millions of air miles can suddenly, for no obvious reason, develop a fear of flying. It doesn't take an accident or a major incident. Anxiety can develop out of nowhere. If flying freaks you out, you are not alone.

It's not all about flying

For those who find flying a terrifying experience, it is worth checking out other causes as well as the direct fear of being involved in a plane crash. If you have a tendency to claustrophobia or vertigo, being in a plane can make these conditions worse. Quite a few fliers find that the confined spaces in aircraft seats and the difficulty of getting out of them make life extremely difficult. Equally, if you suffer from vertigo up a ladder, there's even more opportunity eleven kilometres up in the sky.

For those who hate being hemmed in, an obvious essential is to get yourself an aisle seat. It might also be worth biting the bullet and travelling business class, where the much larger seats feel less confining. The vertigo sufferer needs to work extra hard on distraction and on avoiding views that emphasize the plane's position above the ground. But it is essential to seek medical advice if you suffer from either of these conditions, even though you can take these precautions to minimize the impact of flying.

Mile-high madness

A separate but related issue that has to be faced is the impact of air rage. This is sometimes thought of as a recent phenomenon, but many psychologists suspect that it is the label that is new rather than the condition itself. All the evidence is that the various forms of 'rage' that now trouble us are due to individuals' feeling out of control. The rage response is strongly linked to stress and fear – something that has always been a very common combination in air travel. It is certainly true that there is nothing new about difficult or irrational passengers causing problems for other travellers.

Occasionally the problems can start even before the aircraft is in the air. I was on a flight from London to Paris a number of years ago when we taxied out towards the runway, then, after a short wait, headed back towards the terminal. For a while it wasn't obvious what was happening, but there was obviously something wrong with one of the passengers. Cabin crew were clustered around his seat, arguing with him about something.

Eventually the captain made an announcement. One of the passengers, it seems, was refusing to fasten his seat belt. It was not legally possible for the plane to take off as long as he refused. Quite why the passenger wouldn't take that simple action was never revealed. He may have suffered from claustrophobia. He may simply have been bloody-minded. The crew pointed out to him that they didn't really care about his survival, but it would be unfortunate for the passengers in front if the plane had to stop suddenly and he shot over the seats and decapitated them. Still he refused.

The outcome of this incident was irritating for the passengers – we were delayed for over an hour – but more than irritating for the refusing passenger, who was arrested by police and removed from the plane. He was later fined.

Air rage can produce anything from this form of stress-related irrationality through the boorish behaviour of drunken young travellers to out-and-out violence. Passengers have assaulted cabin crew and fellow passengers for seemingly trivial offences ('the way they spoke to me'). Others have resorted to remarkable behaviour that would normally be associated with urban vandalism, urinating and defecating in the cabin and ripping up seats.

To some extent the present form of air rage seems to have grown as a result of the move of airline travel away from being a luxurious privilege to an everyday form of mass transport that isn't treated much differently from travelling by bus. Passengers don't see why they should obey all the seemingly petty regulations of the airlines that take away their personal control, even if they *are* mostly designed to help them survive, and they get furious. When the restrictions of the regulations are added to the stress that arises from such an unnatural and frightening environment it isn't entirely surprising that rage sometimes boils over.

It is possible that problems with the cabin air (see Chapter 6) are making things worse. Add to this being cooped up in confined conditions and the impact of too much readily available alcohol at an altitude that makes its impact faster and stronger and the stage is set for air rage to be rampant.

Dealing with the rage

It is arguable that airlines could do more to help. They give staff self-defence training and suggestions for restraining unruly passengers, and will refuse flight to someone who is already obviously drunk, but they still continue to pour alcohol as if there is no tomorrow (despite the obvious impact on jet lag even if air rage is ignored) and continue to put marginal earnings above improving air quality and spaciousness of the seats. Perhaps also they should offer free nicotine patches or gum to smokers who are forced (very sensibly) to endure a long flight without a cigarette and inevitably become irritable as their nicotine levels drop.

If you are faced with a fellow passenger who has succumbed to air rage, resist the urge to surge in Rambo-like to try to sort things out. Move away from the person, avoiding eye contact. Look for assistance from the cabin crew. It might be helpful to get the senior crew member, usually called the flight manager or purser, on the case. Give them a clear location and description of what is happening. Try to stay calm. Most cases of air rage can be successfully handled by the cabin crew if they are made aware of the problem as soon as possible.

✈ *Summary:* Flight Stress, Fear of Flying and Air Rage

- It is normal to be afraid of flying.

- The risks of a crash on a particular flight are better than a million to one against.

- Turbulence has hardly ever had a catastrophic effect on a large plane.

- Distraction is essential in dealing with fear and fear-related stress.

- Try simple relaxation techniques.

- Stress can be countered by removing the stressor, or by countering it with physical, emotional and spiritual barriers.

- True fear of flying is a recognized complaint – there are courses available to help.

- If you feel the onset of air rage, use your awareness to control it and keep you safe.

- If you experience air rage in other passengers, don't try to deal with it directly – bring it to the attention of senior cabin crew.

10 On-Board Time Management

Once you are on the plane your options for action are limited. You are confined by your surroundings and the cabin crew's rigid timetable. If you want to make the most of your flight, you need to stay in charge of your time on board.

Even the most seasoned business travellers tend to forget the basics of time management when they get on board an aircraft. It's easy, particularly in business or first class, to let go and give in to the wiles of an impressively high-tech entertainment system. And that's fine if it's what you want to do. But bear in mind that on a long-haul flight you might be spending seven hours, fourteen hours, maybe even as much as twenty-four hours on a plane. That's a serious amount of time to fritter away. In fact, even at the weekend, we never normally have this amount of free time to deal with. There is always something that needs doing.

On the plane, everything is being done by someone else. You are supplementary to requirements, unless you do something about it. And it's important that you do take action – to provide a distraction from any fear you might feel, to take control of your time on board, to use that valuable time and get more enjoyment out of the flight. Given the concerns about health risks, it's all too easy to turn the experience of flying into something like a stay in a hospital ward. There is nothing wrong with making it enjoyable if you can.

→ Fast Track: Balancing Your Time

Spend a moment thinking about the different things you can do on the plane. I'm not suggesting you lay out a detailed agenda, but get a feel for how much of the time you have available you would like to spend on activities under each of these headings:

- Eating

- Working

- Reading

- Using in-flight entertainment (movies, interactive games, audio etc.)

- Using your own entertainment systems (tape-players etc.)

- Sleeping

- Anything else . . .

The M word

We are going to look at each of the ways in which you can spend your time, but first I'd like to spend a moment on that M word in the title of this chapter: management.

I have already emphasized the need to take charge. The single biggest cause of stress is feeling out of control – the more you can make yourself believe that you are in control (whether or not it's true), the less stress you will feel as a result of flying. It's easy to sit back and do as you are told on a flight, but you are surrendering too much if you do.

Have you any choice? After all, the cabin crew are not going to vary their routine to fit in with your wishes, are they? In fact this routine is more under your control the closer you sit to the front of the aircraft – in first class you do get much more freedom to call the shots – but it is true that the crew will never be totally at your beck and call. Yet good management is about making things happen the way you want them to, even if you don't have the authority to order people around. And good management principles can help in getting the best out of the crew.

When you don't have authority you are dependent on an understanding of people to get your way, and it is a matter of simple psychology that you are not going to get the best service if you are surly and rude to the people who are serving you. It is sometimes said that it's a good thing not to be rude to waiters in restaurants in case they spit in your food before they bring it out. Cabin crew may not go to this extreme, but they can certainly make sure that you have an uncomfortable flight if they want to. So why not invest a little effort to make your trip more pleasant?

Perhaps the simplest single thing you can do is to look crew members in the eye and smile when you say thank you for something they have done. It will inevitably have a positive effect, and it will make it easier for them to remember that you are one of the 'good guys' and as such should be given better treatment. It might seem unfair that you have to go to this effort – after all, you have paid your money for your seat and for good service – but remember that cabin crew are human beings who are also suffering all the dehydration, low pressure and other problems associated with flying while trying to give you service.

Combine this simple action with a few other essentials, and you should have the crew on your side. Don't just demand something, explain why you need it (but briefly – the crew are often pressed for time). Be understanding of their pressures – but still ask for what you want. Don't use the call button unless you really have to – catch their eye (remember the smile) or, if they've disappeared, take a stroll and find them. Apologize for disturbing them, even though you are only asking them to do their job. Make them feel good about going out of their way on your behalf.

If you manage to get the crew on your side, they will give you the management role. Rub them up the wrong way and you will get entirely the opposite effect. A valuable example happened to a much-travelled colleague recently. He was flying first class on a transatlantic flight. He was offered a choice of meat or fish for his meal. He pointed out that he was a vegan, and did not want meat, fish or dairy products. The flight attendant told him that it was OK, a vegetarian could eat fish. At this point, my colleague lost his cool.

He told his helpful crew member that, first, vegetarians could not eat fish (though admittedly many people who call themselves vegetarians for convenience of label do). Not only had he been a vegetarian for a long time, but he had been a senior officer of the Vegetarian Society, the body that promotes vegetarianism in the UK. What's more he *wasn't* a vegetarian any more but was now a vegan, with an entirely different requirement. The crew member became flustered and threatened my colleague. She said that if he didn't stop arguing he would be handcuffed for the remainder of the flight and handed over to the NYPD on arrival.

As it happens no action ensued, and my colleague had taken the precaution of recording the conversation from fairly early on, which would have made it difficult for any charges to stick, but it shows that trying to get your way isn't always easy. It is essential not to lose your control. Being confrontational will at best mean that you get no help from the crew, and at worst could result in criminal charges. The crew member's threat was not idle. It is a legal offence to cause a disturbance on an aircraft, and in most circumstances the authorities are more likely to accept the crew member's version of events than your own.

If you want to get your own way in an environment in which the other side has strong powers, politeness and persuasion work better than demanding your rights. I'm not one of these people who thinks that cabin crew are hard done by. (Usually people who do think that way are cabin crew or ex-cabin crew themselves.) No one made them do the job, and most of them enjoy it despite the effort involved. But the fact remains that simple self-interest makes it sensible to go easy on the crew and get them on your side. Once that is achieved, you will have more control of the other aspects of how you spend your time on board. The first, and most pressing, is liable to be if, when and what to eat.

Do I want to eat?

Airline meals are generally full of chemical preservatives. Delivered frozen, they are defrosted with hundreds of other meals in ovens that are cleaned out with chemical products which can get in the food when it is heated. Meals are often served at times that interfere with passengers' attempts to counter jet lag, that disturb sleep, and that encourage indigestion. Does that really sound appealing?

The most important thing to consider when dealing with airline food is timing. A long-distance-traveller friend was flying from Hong Kong to Australia with three companions. Her friends woke her up around two in the morning to tell her that a meal was being served. My friend rather grumpily informed her fellow travellers that she wasn't in the habit of eating at that time and went straight back to sleep. Some airlines are now starting to offer meals in the lounge before flight for business- and first-class passengers who are travelling late (typically on transatlantic routes) – that way you can simply ignore the in-flight catering but not feel that you have missed out.

Airlines serve meals for two reasons: to keep up with the competition (hence all the efforts these days to have meals 'designed' by top chefs) and to keep the passengers under control. If the only imperative were to help passengers to enjoy the flight, the timing of meals would match natural eating patterns. In practice, though, they are timed for the airline staff's convenience and to force passengers into a schedule that works with the flight's timing. A classic example is the evening meal served on the night flights crossing the Atlantic from the USA to Britain. Bearing in mind that once you are on the plane you should be operating on UK time, this is like eating dinner in the middle of the night – not an ideal way to enhance your digestion.

If you want to be in charge, make sure that you eat to suit your needs, not those of the cabin crew. It can be surprisingly hard to say no to free food (or, rather, food that you have unavoidably paid for). But resist. If you aren't hungry, if the meal doesn't fit your destination time, don't eat it. It is much better from a jet-lag viewpoint not to eat at all than to eat at the wrong time. And remember the stress benefits of calling the shots. By taking control of your eating, you are removing one of the potential stressors that can make flying unpleasant and even physically dangerous.

In practice, it shouldn't be that difficult to refuse the meals offered. No matter how they dress it up, airline food is mass-catered fast food. It has to be. There can't be a Michelin-starred kitchen operating out of that tiny galley.

However great the preparation, you are eating the equivalent of reheated convenience food from a supermarket. It might be good convenience food, but that's the limit. What's more, one of the side effects of that cabin air is that your taste buds are less effective. Even if it were a gourmet delight, you couldn't enjoy food on a plane the way you could on the ground.

Quick Tip: Instant Spot Cleaning

Individually packed finger wipes which can be tucked away in your soap bag (and are often provided with an in-flight meal) provide instant spot cleaning for a mark on clothing. This is particularly useful when eating on a plane, as it seems almost impossible to avoid something landing on your clothing.

The wipes are also quite handy before *eating finger food – you can never be quite sure what you have touched on a plane, so it doesn't do any harm to be careful.*

To be fair to the airlines, I have eaten some very good in-flight food (admittedly, mostly during the rare opportunities of experiencing the first-class cabin). I remember some very pleasant roast beef, carved at the seat, and a wonderful pudding with a baked apple surrounded by the most melt-in-the-mouth pastry you could imagine. But that was very much the exception. Most airline meals are high in fat and additives and low in carbohydrates. They aren't too hot on fibre either, but for once this isn't a bad thing. Fibre may be good for your health in general, but it is also a great way to encourage a build-up of gases in the stomach – something you don't want happening with low air pressure.

This lack of carbohydrates (reflecting in part the fact that carbohydrate-rich food tends to be fairly bulky, and bulk is not something an airline galley can accommodate) may be a particular disadvantage, because carbohydrates seem to help you stay alert at a high altitude (many climbers swear by high-carbohydrate diets) by reducing the amount of oxygen required in digestion, and so would help overcome some of the effects of hypoxia.

You could investigate the special-meals options. Some of these are certainly healthier than the typical airline meal – for example, many airlines provide a fruit platter, which is usually quite palatable, contains a lot of water, and doesn't overload your stomach. Equally, some of the alternative meal styles may be higher in carbohydrates than the standard fare. But many special meals are disappointing, with little advantage over the ordinary meals, and of course you do need to order them in advance – typically forty-eight hours before flight. See page 233 for more information.

You may prefer to take your own high-carbohydrate snacks in case you do feel hungry but don't want to indulge in the preservative-rich airline food. UK-based health-food chain Holland & Barrett recommend going for food that is rich in nuts and seeds, or snack foods that are also high in carbohydrates. Be aware, though, that most of these snacks are also quite high in fat. You might be better simply taking a good-quality bread roll.

The soaring office

Work seems a natural way to fill the hours. It certainly isn't impossible to work in the air, though you will find that the reduced oxygen level means a reduction in your usual levels of efficiency. It is best to do the sort of work that you would normally undertake in your 'off' periods during the day, rather than something that requires you to perform at 100 per cent peak efficiency. Admin and routine work are better suited to filling the hours of flight than creative effort. Having said that, creativity guru Edward de Bono completed his book *Six Action Shoes* in the course of a single long flight (and documents his progress through the air as you pass through the book). But this a rare exception to the rule.

If you are going to work in the cabin, you probably want access to all your favourite business tools. Mobile phones are out – they aren't allowed to be used – but many modern planes have 'skyphones' in some seats. These are painfully expensive, but are there if you need an emergency call. Otherwise, you might as well enjoy the rare opportunity to get on with something without constant telephone interruptions.

As for the laptop and the PDA (personal digital assistant – such as a Palm Pilot or a Psion), they're all very well, but I think there's a lot to be said for abandoning your high-tech office and resorting to old-fashioned pen and paper when in the air. The lighting conditions on board are not ideal for computer screens, which can lead to eyestrain. Forcing yourself to take a step away from the keyboard and to use pen and paper can make a refreshing change, giving a different perspective. And, even if you do prefer the laptop at all times, there is considerable confusion over just what is and isn't allowed to be used on a plane.

In part this confusion results from a lack of international standards. The airlines are largely left to set their own policies. My advice is to suppress the mild rage that might arise because the airline is daring to tell you what to do with your own equipment and be overcautious. The concerns about using electronics on board may not have absolute proof attached, but I wouldn't want to risk my life and that of everyone else and the plane just because I couldn't manage without my personal radio.

The problem is that modern planes are highly dependent on sensitive electronics – much more so than the aircraft of forty years ago. All electronic devices are banned from use in the particularly sensitive periods of take-off and landing. Laptops and PDAs are generally thought to be OK otherwise, but I am inclined to give them a miss. All computers give off a fair amount of radio emission, and the only thing that keeps it down is good shielding – I'm not inclined to trust my life to the quality of a computer manufacturer's production line. If you have to use your laptop on board, some airlines can provide power in the business-class seats to keep you operating. However, I have seen a businessman spend a whole flight unsuccessfully trying to get his laptop to charge, so don't depend on this facility.

Settling down with a good book

Although the cabin environment makes it harder to take in information, it is still a great place to just sit and read. Most of us suffer from a lack of time to get into a good book, whether fiction or non-fiction. This enforced spell in an armchair is an excellent opportunity to catch up on some of your reading.

The only restriction I would put on reading material is to keep it easily digestible. This doesn't mean the book has to be lightweight in content, but it should be an easy read. A classical author whose work requires exquisite concentration on each phrase is going to be wasted. You will find that you have skipped whole paragraphs of text without taking them in, or that you get stuck on a line and read it over and over. As long as the book is easy to read – be it a murder mystery, a work of popular science or a business book – it will work fine.

There is also a physical consideration to bear in mind. Great, thick books look tempting, as there's plenty to get through, but they mean a heavy weight in your hand baggage and a heavy weight in your hand as you read. You might be better bringing a number of smaller books rather than a huge doorstop. However, there is one practical advantage – I have found that a very thick omnibus volume containing several novels makes a reasonable footrest if your seat doesn't have one.

IFE

Not long ago, the best in-flight entertainment that the airlines offered was the sight of the cabin crew going through the safety briefing. After that it was all downhill as a scratchy film was projected and you tried to make out the soundtrack through a pair of headphones that resembled a toy stethoscope.

Things have certainly got better. Individual video screens, in the seat backs or on extending supports that unfold from the arms of the seats, give you much more flexibility over choice of movie and TV shows. Some also offer interactive video games and information on the progress of the flight. In business and first class the IFE controller is so complex that I have seen a baffled new flier search confusedly for the button for the reading light for five minutes before the person sitting next to him was kind enough to point it out.

The technology has certainly moved on. Yet we shouldn't be seduced by it. Things still aren't wonderful. Screen size can be small. It's worth asking about this at the time of booking – this is one area where airlines vary considerably. The technology is changing so fast that the relatively slow cycle of aircraft refits will have left some rivals considerably out of date. If your screen is in the seat back, however clever the designer has been, it will be difficult to use if the person in front reclines the seat. And those headphones may be better than they were, but they're still not the same as sitting in front of your stereo system at home.

By all means make use of the in-flight entertainment if you want to, but don't feel obliged to because it's there. I have quite often left my headphones untouched in their wrapper, the screen never activated, without feeling any the worse for it.

Your entertainment systems

In-flight entertainment has certainly improved, but it isn't as flexible as having your own favourite music to hand. Radios are not allowed on board (not that you could get reception at 35,000 ft). Like radio-controlled toys and mobile phones, they are banned as a possible safety risk. The crucial measure of safeness is whether or not a product gives off electromagnetic radiation – radio waves, for example. Unfortunately, you can't always rely on common sense to identify just what is safe in this respect. For example, all radio receivers give off some radio waves as well as picking up your favourite station.

There is less agreement on CD players, which are banned by some airlines and not by others. A friend who spends most of his time jetting around the world swears by his mini-disc player, which he carries along with a compact music library in his briefcase. Some airlines will let him use it, some won't. There's more general agreement that tape players are OK, so you shouldn't have any trouble with your Walkman, even if the sound quality isn't quite as good.

If you prefer something more interactive, hand-held

games machines are generally considered acceptable as well (if you can face sitting next to someone while wrestling with Super Puzzle Fighter II on your Gameboy). Personally, despite being told that hand-held games are safe from the radio-emission viewpoint, I would even be suspicious of them, as they must carry some form of processor and a timing oscillator. I have heard engineers cast doubts on the impact that most electronic goods can have – but they usually have their feet planted safely on the ground at the time. The chances of a problem arising may be remote, but I don't want to risk my life on even a remote possibility if it can be avoided. And, of course, whatever the device, don't use it during take-off and landing.

Anything else...

Although the physical layout of the aircraft places restrictions on you, remember that you are not welded to your seat. It's to your benefit to get up and have a wander, if only to reduce the risk of deep-vein thrombosis. But you can also find some entertainment in simply taking a look around the most expensive vehicle you are ever likely to travel in.

There may not be a gym on board (yet), but you can take the opportunity of moving around to indulge in a little discreet exercising. Perhaps the best place to do this is in the toilet. Although the space is restricted, at least you can do your running on the spot or knee bends without feeling foolish.

At one time, this was also the site of an alternative type of exercise. A former stewardess with BOAC has told me that it was possible on some early aircraft to unscrew the panel between two adjacent toilets to make it possible to discreetly become a member of the Mile High Club (there was also more space that way). Frankly, most aircraft toilets are not the most romantic of locations, even if they might throw in a small flower arrangement up the front. Better to stick to more solitary forms of exercise on board.

You might also take the opportunity of the unusual amount of free time to indulge yourself spiritually. If you are in the habit of praying or meditating, here is a rare chance to do so without having to worry about the next thing you have to do. It sounds corny, but it really is possible to turn the problem of what to do with all that time into an opportunity. With the right time management, the hours will drop away. Before long, you will need to consider your destination.

The arrival-airport blues

Although most of us feel a sense of relief when the aircraft eventually touches down safely at our destination, the roar of the reverse thrust dies down, and we begin the long taxi to the stand, the journey isn't quite over. We still have the arrival airport to get through and the journey to our final destination.

Keep your wits about you. The signing in a strange airport may be different to the familiar signs back home.

Don't rely too much on the sheep syndrome, following the passengers in front of you – someone up front could be lost. Keep an eye on the signs, and be prepared to do things your way.

Be particularly wary at immigration and customs. Most airports will have different immigration desks for local passport holders and others – make sure you know which queue to be in. When you get near to the immigration desk, look out for lines painted on the floor. It is common practice to expect passengers to wait behind a line until the desk is ready for them. While you are unlikely to be shot for breaking this rule, I have seen some immigration officials and guards become surprisingly threatening to passengers who get it wrong.

As well as your passport, the immigration officials in most countries will expect a form to have been filled out by any foreign nationals. This should have been given you on the plane. All too often I have seen people thrown to the back of an immigration queue because they have forgotten to fill out the form. The best approach is to fill it out as soon as you are given it and tuck it away in your passport.

Having recovered your bags (if there are any problems, see page 247), you will need to pass through customs. Again, don't assume that the familiar rules apply. Check the boards showing the amounts you can bring in through customs, even if you looked it up before you left home. (The rules might have changed.) If there is any doubt, it isn't worth taking a risk – don't go for the green channel.

If your bags do need to be examined, open them yourself. Make it easy for the customs official. I have seen it suggested that you can deter customs officials in Japan from going through your luggage by putting dirty underwear at the top. It is possible this may work, but I wouldn't rely on it. Be aware of the very strong penalties for importing drugs into some countries. In some parts of the world, drug smuggling carries a mandatory death penalty. Don't take the risk.

Quick Tip: **Keep Those Tags**

Don't rip off your baggage tags as soon as you arrive at the airport. Leave them on until you've had a chance to check your luggage and its contents. It's time to get rid of them once you are sure you won't need to make a claim. If you do find something wrong, ring the airline immediately, keep a note of who you speak to and when you made the call, and see page 257 for more advice.

Once you are out into the airport concourse, if you aren't being met you will probably want a taxi. Some major hotels run shuttle buses – it's worth checking to see if one of these is available. If you do need a taxi, don't allow yourself to be led off by a tout. Look for the airport's official taxi line, which will usually be controlled. If it isn't obvious, ask at an information desk. Check with the taxi driver what the fare will be before getting in.

✈ *Summary:* On-Board Time Management

- Have a rough plan to make use of your time.

- Take control of the cabin crew by effective management.

- Eat only if you want to, and stick to light, high-carbohydrate meals.

- By all means work, but don't try to do 'high-concentration' work.

- Try using pen and paper for a refreshing change from the computer.

- Make use of the time to rediscover reading.

- Be selective about in-flight entertainment.

- Bring your own entertainment systems, but be very wary of any interference dangers.

- Take a look around and get some exercise.

- Make use of the opportunity for prayer or meditation if either appeals.

11 Flying with Kids

Even regular business travellers sometimes fly with children, and most of us with families are going to experience the delights of a holiday flight with the kids along. Making the experience of flying safe for our children (and bearable for us) isn't just a matter of buying them a ticket. It helps to consider the physiological differences between children and adults – and their different needs and approach to life.

We all know how children make everything take longer, whether it's getting into the car for a journey or getting packed to go on holiday. Taking children on a flight will mean more preparation, but it will be worth it if you can reduce the stress they cause. Sometimes they may have to face a journey by air alone, and then even more than usual you need to be prepared.

Booking the kids

Airports and planes are potentially dangerous environments. You will want to make sure that you keep your children with you at all times. This can sometimes be easier said than done – unfortunately, families quite often turn up at the airport only to find that they are unable to sit together on the plane. When you make a reservation with children, make it clear that you are a family and ask for a note to be made to try to ensure that you are seated together. If the worst comes to the worst and you end up seated apart on the plane, tell the cabin crew. If approached sympathetically they will often try to arrange a swap of seats before take-off, and will always make an attempt once the seat-belt signs are off.

A few other things to consider when you are booking. Will you want children's meals or baby food (see page 233)? Can you find a non-stop flight to your destination? This is particularly valuable – not only will you save a couple of hours, you will miss out on the nightmare of trying to cross a transit airport with one or more children in tow. As you will know, children are difficult to hurry at the best of times, and trying not to miss a plane in a strange airport is anything but the best of times.

Remember too, when you are booking, that the selection of when you are going to fly will influence your comfort on board. Ideally you'd like plenty of room on the plane. It will make it easier for your children to stretch out and take a nap, and they are less likely to be sick over the business-man in the next seat. The obvious times to miss are around holidays, like just before Christmas. You can also miss weekly and daily rushes by avoiding the 'business times' – to have the best chance of some extra space, try for midweek, and for flights that either leave very early or around the middle of the day.

Children are people too

Don't assume that, because they aren't adults, your children won't need the appropriate paperwork. In the UK, children now have to have their own passports (though they can remain on an existing parental passport until it expires). Bizarrely, this means having to take a passport photograph even of small babies, and the same Byzantine regulations apply as for adult photos – so you can't be in the photograph holding your baby.

Quick Tip: Use a Pro

Many professional photographers have equipment that enables them to take passport-approved photographs. Rather than struggle with keeping your baby in place on the precarious stool of an automatic photo booth while the photograph is taken, consider using a photographer, who will be able to seat your baby in a safer location.

If you are determined to do it yourself with the booth, make sure you use one of the more modern variety which lets you see the photo before you print it. The chances are that you will need several attempts to get an acceptable shot.

Check all the same requirements that you would for an adult (see page 31), like visas and inoculations. It is particularly important to check with your doctor about the medical implications of any countries with special requirements, as some conditions are much more dangerous for children.

Suffer the little children

If you are a defensive parent, you may find that the attitude of other passengers towards your children seems negative. It is, however, possible to have a degree of sympathy with their viewpoint. These people have paid a lot of money to go through a very stressful experience. It will not be helped by having yoghurt poured all over them, or by having a constant piercing scream echoing in their already suffering ears.

Resist the temptation to demand your parental rights. It may well have been your lack of preparation that precipitated any problems. You need to keep your children entertained and occupied. This means bringing enough books, games, puzzles and other entertainment to last through the flight. When it comes to feeding time, try to ensure that you are there as a buffer between your children and other passengers. If it means reducing the chances of being covered in food, most passengers will be willing to move in order to accommodate you.

If you want to get cooperation and a positive response from those around you, be prepared to be manipulative. Dress your small children in their Sunday best, and keep them as clean as you can. That way, even if they are crying, they will seem a lot more attractive than a toddler covered in food with a runny nose. You may well get more help and attention from the cabin crew too. Many crew members have children of their own and can be very helpful – as long as they feel they can come close to your child without getting their uniform soiled. Of course it's not always easy, but it is worth making an extra effort for the sympathy vote.

Little bodies

Newborns under ten to twelve weeks old should not travel, as the airways of the lungs might not be fully developed, causing distress when air pressure goes down. In a 1998 *British Medical Journal* article it was reported that a number of newborn babies had died within a day or two of flying. While there was not conclusive proof of a cause, it was thought that the reason had been the effect of the lowered air pressure on the infants' underdeveloped lungs. Taking a very young baby on an aircraft, except in a dire emergency, should be considered an unacceptable risk.

All children up to their late teens have a higher body-water content than adults, and as a result are more vulnerable to dehydration. They should be given small amounts of water at frequent intervals. Even more so than with adults, it is essential to carry your own bottled water for this. Don't give way to pressure to substitute fizzy drinks, which might result in indigestion in the pressurized cabin. Particularly avoid colas, which are diuretics, effectively squeezing water out of the cells and encouraging dehydration.

We have already seen how the child's smaller Eustachian tube makes the impact of pressure changes on the ear more painful (see page 113). Small children also find it harder to make small corrections to the pressure balance by swallowing or yawning. To reduce the onset of painful ears, try using a dummy (a 'pacifier' in the USA) for smaller children, or getting an older child to suck a boiled sweet.

→ Fast Track:
Basic Child Comfort

- Babies under around twelve weeks can suffer from breathing problems – if at all possible, don't fly with them.

- Children have a higher water content and dehydrate easier than adults – keep up the water consumption.

- Avoid fizzy drinks and colas.

- Explain the need to yawn and swallow to correct pressure in the ears.

- Use a dummy (pacifier) for very small children, or sucking a hard sweet for older ones, to help correct air-pressure differences.

To seat, or not to seat

For the first two years of your child's flying life you have an important choice to make. The airline will let infants under the age of two travel without a seat. If you go for this option, your child will be able to fly for between nothing and 10 per cent of the full fare, as against between a quarter and a half of the fare to get him or her a seat. To earn this saving you will have to hold the child in your lap during take-off and landing. But is this really what you want?

Think through the length of your flight with a baby wedged on your knees. OK, there may be spare seats, but you certainly can't guarantee it. Long-haul flights seem long enough as it is – with a baby permanently installed they can become an eternity. Think of meals and getting to the toilet. Think of changing your baby and settling him or her down to sleep. There is another consideration too. The only reason you won't have booked a seat was to cut the cost of flying. But would you let your baby travel loose in your car without a safe car seat just to save money?

By not having a seat you will certainly save on airfare. But there is no doubt at all that, in the event of a crash, you will have reduced your child's chance of survival to almost zero. He or she will also be at more risk of being hurt or killed if there is severe turbulence. It is still a decision that has to be made. As we will see in Chapter 15, crashes are very unusual. But be aware of what you are doing in making that decision.

If you do decide to carry a baby or toddler on your lap, make sure that you are sitting in a row with an extra oxygen mask, in case of emergencies. You can't share a mask with your baby, and both of you will need the oxygen. Usually the rows with spare masks are at the front of each section, but check with the cabin crew to make sure. There is only one extra mask, so be sure to ask for assistance if you find yourself in a row with another child on a lap.

During take-off and landing with a baby on your lap, get a clip-on supplementary belt if they are available. They won't stand up to a crash, but they will help if it's bumpy. Hold the baby firmly against your chest with your arms crossed around his or her back. Don't try to fasten your seat belt around the baby – it could cause serious harm if there is a sudden jerk.

You will also need to make sure that there are enough laps available to accommodate your young travellers. I have seen parents turn up at an airport with three small children and be surprised that they weren't allowed on the flight. If there are fewer of you than there are lap children, you will only be able to travel if you find another passenger kind enough to have a strange baby on his or her lap.

If you do give a child a seat of his or her own – and I can't recommend this strongly enough – use a safety seat with it if you would normally expect to use a safety seat in a car. Small children cannot be effectively secured by an adult's lap belt. A child seat may be a hassle, but it does add much more safety.

The American Federal Aviation Authority strongly recommends that all children who fly, regardless of their age, make use of a restraint appropriate to their size and weight. A good rule of thumb is to use a child seat for children weighing less than 18 kg (and a special, backward-facing baby seat under around 9 kg). Some airlines will provide child seats – check when you make your reservation. This is obviously the best option if available, as it will save you from carrying around a seat – often a cumbersome device, and especially challenging if you have to make a connection mid-route. If you do ask the airline to supply a seat, confirm this before flight and at the check-in desk.

If you take your own seat with you, check with the airline that it is happy with this, and make sure that the seat can be secured with a lap belt only. You will also need to be sure that your seat fits in the relatively small width of an aircraft seat. Most economy seats will take a child seat no wider than about 40 cm, but ask your airline for details.

Your child should be allocated a window seat, as safety regulations usually preclude the use of child seats away from the window, to stop them getting in the way of an evacuation. For the same reason, they can't be used in exit rows.

Even if your baby or toddler has a seat, you might want it to spend part of the flight on your lap. You can get hold of special safety garments that keep the child safe in the event of turbulence (see page 326). These usually consist of some form of harness that is attached to your seat belt. Note that these safety garments are not allowed to be used during take-off and landing. This same ban applies to strap-on baby carriers and booster seats – the special cushions quite often used in cars when children are too big for child seats but too small to use the normal seat belt unaided.

Some airlines will provide a small cot for young babies to use during the main part of the flight. These are typically around 70 by 30 cm in size, so will only do for babies under around 5 kg. Check with your airline at reservation whether a cot can be provided – if it can, you will need to reserve it then, and it's worth ringing a couple of days before departure to ensure it is going to be available.

Little appetites

If you are travelling with a fussy baby, take along his or her favourite food. Even if your little darling will eat anything and everything, don't assume that the airline will carry baby food on board. Many don't provide for babies at all. Even airlines that do supply baby food probably won't have much or any available just in case. Treat it as a special meal (see page 233), requesting it at reservation and checking before departure. And even then I would take some food with you. No one wants to risk spending hours on a long flight with a hungry baby.

Make sure that you order a child's meal for toddlers and above. If an adult's meal is served on the flight, the chances are the children won't like it. Airline kids' meals may be just as unimaginative as the sort of thing you get in a pub – sausages, burgers, chicken nuggets – but at least they should get a positive reaction. Once your children reach that difficult stage when it's not cool to be a kid (you'll know if they are there), don't embarrass them by labelling them children in this way. If your children have reached this stage but still won't like airline food, ask them to pack something for themselves.

For any age of child, though, it's best to carry a supply of snacks with you. If the airline does serve food it might not be at the right time, and the chances are your offspring will be hungry more often than the trolley will provide for. You could leave home early in the day and get to your departure late and never get a decent meal out of the airline. Keep the snacks light, with plenty of carbohydrates – plain poppadams, for instance, are great.

Bearing in mind the need to keep your child from dehydration, take plenty of bottled water. The tap water on an aircraft isn't recommended drinking for anyone, and especially not babies and children, who may be more susceptible to the water-treatment chemicals and any bugs that are present. That same bottled water needs to be used to make up any diluted drinks or formula milk. Cabin crew should be able to use a jug of hot water to get a bottle up to temperature if your baby needs a warmed bottle. There aren't microwave ovens on planes for safety reasons, so that's the best you'll get.

There are mixed feelings about breast-feeding a baby on an aircraft. There are no medical reasons why you shouldn't, but it remains a fact that breast-feeding embarrasses many people. The reaction you are likely to get varies from country to country – European passengers are less likely to react badly than US ones, for example. If you get a window seat and there's no one seated next to you, there is no reason at all why anyone should have a problem with it. You may well argue that there's no reason, full stop, why anyone else should have a problem with you breast-feeding, but the fact is that some do. An aircraft seat in a crowded plane puts you much closer to a stranger than you would normally be, and this does make it too intimate an act for many.

Forty winks

The good news is that the noise of a plane's engines is even better at getting children off to sleep than a car, so if you are in the habit of taking your little ones on a quick tour of the countryside to get them to drop off you should find they sleep pretty easily. If you sit in the rear half of the plane, behind the wings, there will be a little more engine noise, which can be beneficial rather than negative in this case.

Some parents, desperate to get their children to drop off, use antihistamines and other non-prescription drugs that have a tendency to induce drowsiness. This is not a remedy I would recommend, and it certainly shouldn't be used unless experience on the ground has shown it to be effective – it actually makes some children more active. It's much better if their sleep can be natural.

Nappy rash

If your child is still in nappies, at some point in a long flight you are going to have to make the change. Don't try to do this on the floor of the aircraft – you don't know what has been spilled down there. If there is plenty of space, it is probably best to do it on an empty seat (well away from other passengers' noses). Make sure you keep a hand on the baby's body throughout the change, as a sudden jolt could send him or her flying. As changing nappies some-times seems to require you to grow a third arm anyway, adding the need to pin your baby down means it's a lot easier if you've a partner along to help.

When the old nappy is off you can fold it tightly and push it into one of the sickbags from the seat pockets in front of you. Don't ask the cabin crew to dispose of it – they aren't allowed to, because they handle food. Instead, take it along to the toilet and hope that the disposal bin isn't already full. Don't try to get it down the toilet itself – aircraft toilets aren't designed for large objects.

If there aren't enough empty seats, you will have to make the change in the confined space of the toilet. Some planes now have a pull-down changing surface, but it's still pretty fiddly and you will still need to have an extra hand to keep your baby safe. Alternatively you can sit on the toilet seat and try to make the change in your lap. It's not exactly easy, but at least it's a way to while away a few minutes. Keep the baby's head towards you, so there isn't going to be a head-first fall on the floor if he or she manages to wiggle out of your grip.

It is, in principle, possible for two of you to manage the operation in the toilet, but it's cramped to say the least. The best bet if you want to try this is to leave the door open, but watch out for passing trolleys.

Packing for children

There's a difficult balance to be achieved when packing an in-flight bag for a trip with children. On the one hand you need to be able to cope with the worst possible case, when you are delayed and your bags get lost. On the other hand the last thing you want is a bulky, heavy bag to manage as well as your screaming infant. Some form of backpack is the best way to carry all those little essentials.

You are going to need to carry at least one change of clothes per child. In theory it's also a good idea to take a swimming costume and towel – if you turn up in a strange place without bags, you can at least keep your child occupied by spending time in the pool. In practice, you might decide to take the risk and buy costumes and towels on the spot rather than burden yourself with these heavy items.

Absolutely essential, though, are snacks, activities, games and toys. And if your child has any irreplaceable toy – perhaps a cuddly bunny or a blanket without which he or she can't go to sleep – make sure you keep that with you at all times. You can't afford to lose this with the checked-in luggage.

Once your children can manage it, let them have backpacks of their own. It will keep the weight down in your bag, and they will enjoy the chance of some independence. Let them decide what will go in the bag (perhaps with a little guidance), and make sure they pack the day before, so you can all be happy they can carry it.

With babies and toddlers you are going to have more to carry. By all means take a pushchair to reduce the strain, but don't take a heavy-duty cross-country model. If necessary, it is probably worth buying a small, cheap pushchair that folds away like an umbrella, as you should be able to get it in an overhead locker. Go with a big buggy and it is going to end up as hold baggage – which means you don't get the benefit on the long trek to the departure gate.

→ Fast Track:
Baby and Toddler Packing Guide

- Bottles

- Nappies

- Wipes

- Cream

- Damp facecloths in plastic bags

- Bottled water (lots)

- Formula milk

- Baby food

- Snacks in small portions

- Teething biscuits and gel

- Clean clothes for both of you

- Juice and milk in boxes

- Trainer cups

- Dummy

- Favourite cuddly

- Soft, lightweight blankets

- Any medication

- Freshen-up kit for you

Getting through the flight

Bear in mind that you are responsible for your child while on board, not the cabin crew. They may be prepared to help out in quiet times, but you can't depend on it. Although your child is not going to open a door and fall out (it's physically impossible in a pressurized cabin), there are plenty of hazards around the aircraft, particularly if he or she should stray into the galley. You are most vulnerable at times when you may fall asleep. If you are travelling alone with a small child, make sure that you take some form of restraint that prevents the child from wandering too far away without your knowledge.

Quick Tip: **The Joys of Novelty**

A long-term airline employee and regular flier with two children suggests that the best survival aid for a long flight with children is novelty. 'Take along a bag stuffed with small things that are new to the child. It doesn't have to cost much, but novelty counts for a lot, particularly with young children. If they can spend the journey making small discoveries it will be beneficial for both you and them.'

In theory the best place for a child is sandwiched between two responsible adults, but the main requirement is to try to keep him or her away from other passengers and out of danger. It's best not to put a child in an aisle seat, where the close-moving, heavy trolleys can trap little fingers. In practice, most children will desperately want a window seat, and there's no good reason to deprive them

---

Quick Tip: **Mystery Tour**

With a little preparation you can provide older children with an on-board mystery to solve. Take a prepared book, or use an in-flight magazine to provide the answers to a quiz, organized into the framework of a short adventure story.

For example, using an in-flight magazine, you could pretend that the child is a spy. He or she has to find a route (using the route maps) from (say) London to Sydney taking in every continent except Antarctica. Additional tasks are to find at least three fascinating facts about a capital city, the name of the editor of the magazine, and the name of someone who runs a museum, art gallery or restaurant, and also to draw a map to get from the aircraft to the exit of the destination airport. (These questions will have to fit the content of the magazine.) The spy's expenses will be equal to the sum of the prices of the three most expensive bottles of spirits for sale in the in-flight shop, and . . . you could carry on indefinitely. Make sure there are little prizes available.

---

of the experience. If you are using a child seat, using the window position will be an essential.

Consider the limitations of the space when you bring items on board to keep your child entertained. Think what he or she really plays with, and the amount of space taken up in the process. Go for popular, low-space activities. The airline may well provide something, but don't expect much more than a colouring book and crayons – even so, it will probably go down well because it is associated with the special time of being on an aircraft, so always ask. A particularly friendly cabin-crew member may even be able to find a pack of cards with the airline logo on the back. In principle these are for sale, but there is often a discretionary pack that can be given away.

→ Fast Track:
Entertainment Pack

Making the trip endurable means keeping the children entertained while minimizing the disruption to everyone else on the plane. Avoid toys that are going to make you cringe.

	Types of toy	Examples
Avoid:	Noisy toys, toys that squirt water, toys that scatter mess across the floor, electronic toys (see page 197)	Talking toys, talking books, sound-effect guns and vehicles, water pistols, water toys, glitter art, paint sets, gunk

Take for babies:	Toys you would attach to a pram or pushchair, toys that can be chewed, manipulated or (quietly) rattled, visually interesting objects, objects with different touch sensations	Plastic keys, cuddly toys, mirror toys, baby books, hand puppets, woollen pompom, unbreakable 'snowfall' paperweight. You are probably the best toy of all for a baby, and will need to animate the other toys
Take for toddlers:	Individual small toys (some new) wrapped in small bags, books, drawing materials, manipulation toys	Keys, contents of your handbag, purse or wallet, cuddly toys, board books, tell-the-time books, pop-up books, picture books, small but chunky cars, dolls and animals, scribbling pad and coloured crayons
Take for older children:	Individual small toys (some new), wrapped in small bags, books, drawing materials, games, imaginary-play toys	Reading books, audiobooks, sticker books, colouring and drawing books with crayons, dot-to-dot pictures, pencil mazes, puzzle books, playing cards, travel games, small figures, animals, dolls and cars, fuzzy felt, tapestry kit, hand-held maze games, family photo album, puzzles, small Lego sets, cat's-cradle string and instructions

Away from home alone

Occasionally it may be necessary for one or more of your children to travel on their own. The large airlines are very good at handling 'UMs' (unaccompanied minors), and will make sure they are well supervised. However, the airline's responsibility ceases as soon as it hands over the child at the destination.

It is essential that you give clear details of who is going to pick up the child, and that that same person turns up at the destination, complete with effective means of identification. You will also want to give the airline contact details both for the destination and for where you can be reached, in case, for whatever reason, your designated person doesn't show up.

When you drop off the child, allow time to stay at the airport until you can be sure that the plane has taken off. And of course take the obvious precautions of giving the child suitable ID and a stronger than usual lecture on not going anywhere with strangers. Unaccompanied children can hardly avoid talking to strangers under the circumstances, but you can get them to stick to airline staff.

→ Fast Track: Unaccompanied Minors

- Book only non-stop flights with no connections if possible.

- Make sure that the child is enrolled in the airline's frequent-flier scheme. Some airlines have special children's schemes with appropriate benefits.

- If booking by phone, advise the agent of the child's age and ask exactly what will be done to help.

- If booking online, phone up afterwards to do the same.

- Ask for a window seat – your child will appreciate it, and he or she is less likely to wander round the aircraft.

- Order a special child's meal (ideally forty-eight hours in advance – see page 233).

- If this is your child's first flight, ask it to be noted in the PNR (Passenger Name Record).

- Let both the airline and the child know who will be picking him or her up.

- If the person doing the pickup changes, you must let the airline know – it can't release the child to anyone else.

- Give the child some cash for headphones or phone calls, or to buy food in case of a delay. Let him or her know what is free and what will have to be paid for.

- Don't book your child on the last flight of the evening unless it is unavoidable, to minimize the chance of being left behind after a cancellation.

- Don't leave the airport until the plane has taken off – if the passengers have to come back for any reason, you want to be there for your child.

- Pin a note to the child's clothing with details of the trip, contact names and numbers, and any allergies or special medicines required.

- Remind the person doing the picking-up to bring good identification.

- Make sure that the child knows how to ring you, including any dialling codes that might apply.

- Reinforce the usual message about not going off with strangers.

Travelling with children is never going to be as easy as travelling on your own, but it doesn't have to be a nightmare. There are some plus points. If you are scared of flying, you will find that the need to give your children attention will provide a very effective distraction once the take-off is over. And there is something infectious about the excitement and wonder that children experience – they are yet to become cynical, experienced fliers.

The single biggest factor that will influence the success of your journey is how much you prepare. Even if you hate making lists and being organized, this is one time when thinking through every aspect of the journey and putting extra effort into packing the right things will pay you back one-hundredfold.

✈ *Summary:* Flying with Kids

- Plan!

- Remember that passports, visas and immunization apply to children as well as to adults.

- Some of the effects of flight, such as low air pressure

and dehydration have more effect on children. Take account of this.

- Give serious consideration to getting a seat even for a baby, and use a child seat for any child too small to cope with a normal seat belt.

- Be prepared for feeding your child – don't expect the airline to do everything.

- Take plenty of snacks and bottled water.

- Provide entertainment – pack appropriate toys and games.

- Let older children fill their own small backpack (with a little parental filtering if necessary).

- If sending a child unaccompanied, make sure the collector has appropriate documentation.

12 The Special-Needs Traveller

Although the airlines and airports will claim to be doing their best for those with special needs – from travellers requiring a vegetarian diet to those needing wheelchair access – at times it seems that they are hiding behind safety and engineering issues to avoid taking the trouble to make life easier for these passengers. If you have special needs, you will have to accept some restrictions – occupants of seats in escape rows, for example, have to be readily mobile and capable of moving a heavy emergency-exit door. Other aspects of the airline experience should be capable of more flexibility to fit with your requirements.

At the airport

The airline will usually provide some assistance in getting to and from the plane and in making a connection, but won't be able to provide full-time assistance when at the gate – if you need this, you will have to travel with a companion. It will also provide transfers on and off the planes, using special wheelchairs designed for aircraft aisles.

Transport to and from the gate can potentially be made using electric buggies or the airline's or your own wheelchair, but if your own wheelchair is in the hold it may not be practicable to get it out and assembled until after arrival. If you are in a hurry it might be better to take an airline chair and pick up your own at baggage collection. Unfortunately there can also be considerable delays when waiting for an airline wheelchair to arrive. In the short term it makes sense to allow extra time at the airport and for connections – but also lobby the airline for better support.

Most flights now make use of air bridges to allow flat access to the aircraft door, but at some airports it is still necessary to use steps. If you can't manage these, it is important to let the airline know at the time of booking (and again forty-eight hours before flying) so that alternative arrangements can be made. These will usually require you to board and disembark a significant time before or after the other passengers.

Aircraft features

Airlines are getting better at disabled access inside aircraft, but it takes a long time to refit the entire fleet of a major carrier. Depending on the age and type of your aircraft, you may find facilities like movable aisle armrests, wheelchair stowage, on-board wheelchairs, and wheelchair-accessible toilets (these last tend to be practicable only on larger aircraft).

If you are likely to need a seat with a movable armrest to

make it easier to get from a chair in the aisle into the seat, let the airline know at the time of your reservation. Bring this up again at check-in and at the gate. If you arrive on the plane and find you haven't got one, let the cabin crew know. They will do their best, but if they have unexpectedly been allocated an aircraft that doesn't have movable aisle armrests there is nothing they can do about it.

Wheelchair assault course

Wheelchair users can rightly feel that they are getting a raw deal. Only a few days ago I heard a wheelchair athlete complain about being told she would have to give up her wheelchair at check-in. She pointed out that it felt to her as it might to some of the other passengers if they were asked to take off their shoes and socks before checking in.

That said, on a particular day you will have to live with the provision that has been made for wheelchair-handling in the airport and on the aircraft. Whether or not you can keep your own wheelchair will depend on a number of factors.

Some airlines make provision for on-board stowage of a personal wheelchair. Usually there is space for only one chair, allocated on a first come, first served basis. If you want to get that space you will need to make sure you book early. You will also probably have to arrive at the airport in time to be one of the first on board the aircraft. Your chair will have to fit into the storage area and be of an appropriate weight – the airline will let you know the limitations.

If your chair is electrically powered, you must ensure that you have a gel or dry-cell battery. Wet-cell batteries (like a car battery) contain corrosive acids that can cause serious damage to aircraft and put the passengers at risk. They are not allowed in the cabin or loose in the hold. If you are dependent on using a wet-cell battery, it can be shipped in the hold with special packaging, but the airline will need at least forty-eight hours' warning and you will have to allow at least an hour at the airport for the battery to be packed away.

If you can't (or don't want to) take your personal wheelchair on board, there will usually be one provided by the airline. This will be specially designed to fit in the aisle of the aircraft, and can be useful not only to get to your seat but also to get to the toilet. Cabin crew should know how to operate the wheelchair and will help with its use, but aren't required to lift or carry you.

Canes and crutches

Canes and crutches can be taken on board, but their size and capabilities will determine exactly how they can be stored. Telescopic canes can be tucked away in the seat back or your hand baggage. If this is not possible, you can store canes and crutches in an approved cupboard or baggage-stowage area (this does not include the toilets), in the overhead bins or under the seats, provided they don't protrude into the aisle or block an emergency row. Under the seat, canes have to be laid flat on the floor.

Usually canes and crutches can be accommodated, but think through your particular items and where they are going to go. If in doubt, ask beforehand – don't turn up on the day and get a nasty surprise.

Canes need to be stowed during take-off and landing – visually impaired travellers should ask cabin crew for an explanation of emergency procedures and aircraft surroundings during the flight.

Special in-flight needs

On board the aircraft, the crew will be able to help in a number of areas, but bear in mind that they often have to deal with a considerable number of passengers in a short time, and that there are some restrictions placed on the help they can offer. If you need more assistance you will have to take along a companion (ensure that you are seated together by emphasizing his or her role at booking and check-in).

It is reasonable to expect help from the cabin crew in dealing with an on-board wheelchair, in stowing and retrieving items from lockers and under the seat, in identifying food items on your meal tray, and in opening packages for you. However, crew are not permitted to help with feeding, personal hygiene and using the toilet. They cannot lift you or provide medical services like giving injections.

Guide dogs and other animals

If you have a guide dog or other animal that is trained to help you with mobility, visual or hearing difficulties it will normally be accepted in the aircraft cabin without charge.

The animal will have to occupy the floor space where you sit, and will not be allowed to obstruct the aisle or any route for emergency evacuation. Bear in mind that any such animal will be subject to the quarantine and pet-passport restrictions of any foreign country you are visiting – and of your own country on your return. See page 241 for details.

Medication

Never put medication in checked luggage in the hold – always include it in your hand baggage. That way you will always have access to it in an emergency, and it is much less likely to go missing. Bear in mind that planes do not usually have on-board fridges that can be used to store temperature-sensitive medicines – you will need to take your own precautions if necessary.

If your medication involves the use of needles, get a letter from your doctor specifying the requirement. This can be helpful if security or customs have queries. The last thing you want is to be held up by an official in a foreign country who suspects you of travelling with illegal drugs or with a form of weapon.

If you have a drip or other intravenous device that needs

to be hung up, bear in mind that this can't be done in a normal aircraft seat, as it might interfere with on-board emergency oxygen masks. In some seats you may be able to have such a device as long as you can handle a separate oxygen cylinder – alternatively, you may need to use an extremely expensive air ambulance.

Access to oxygen

If you need medical oxygen supplies, you will not be allowed to bring your own oxygen bottle on board. You must ask the airline to provide one – and give it at least forty-eight hours' notice to do this. There will be a charge for the provision. The airline will expect to get a certificate from your doctor specifying your need for oxygen and the appropriate flow rate. This will normally be accepted at check-in. Although aircraft do all carry emergency oxygen bottles, they cannot be used for a known requirement.

If you want to take your own oxygen bottles along with you, they can be stored in checked baggage as long as they are completely empty and depressurized. This is an essential requirement – a pressurized bottle that is not specially designed for the aircraft environment could blow out, ripping open the side of the aircraft and causing a crash.

The airline will normally provide oxygen only for inflight use. You will need to make your own arrangements if you need oxygen at the airport. Remember that this will include any connecting airports.

Other assistive devices

You are allowed to bring other life-support and assistance devices on board as long as they do not involve pressurized equipment. Typical examples are respirators, nebulizers and ventilators. However, if it won't fit in the normal storage, you will be required to purchase an extra seat for the equipment. As with wheelchairs, you will not be allowed any equipment that is powered by wet-cell batteries – make sure that your equipment runs from dry-cell or gel batteries. Few planes can provide an electrical supply, so you will probably be dependent on batteries.

→ Fast Track:
   Medical Certificates

If you suffer from certain conditions, you will need to obtain a medical certificate from your doctor within ten days of flight, and let the airline know at check-in. Note that a certificate does not guarantee that you will be allowed to fly by the airline, nor does it mean that you are fit to fly (see page 36). You will need a medical certificate if you:

- need medical oxygen – the certificate must state your need for oxygen and the required flow rate;

- have a communicable disease or infection – the certificate must state any conditions or precautions that must be taken to avoid transmission of the condition; or

- have a medical condition where there is reasonable doubt that you can complete the flight safely without requiring medical assistance during the flight.

Eating to order

If you have special meal requirements, make sure that you let the airline know at least forty-eight hours before travelling. And keep telling it. Reconfirm your requirements a day before leaving home. Make sure at check-in. This may seem like overkill, but even the best airlines have a tendency to slip up on special meals. You could check once you are on board as well, though by then the chances are that there is nothing that can be done about it if your requirement hasn't been loaded.

A useful aid, especially if you want one of the more unusual special meals, is to be aware of the international meal codes used by the airlines (see Fast Track – Special Meal Types). To maximize the chances of getting your required meal, specify the code as well as the type. It's all too easy, for example, for someone to hear 'vegetarian' when they're told 'vegan'. Check that the correct meal type appears in your confirmation and on your ticket or itinerary.

This preparation is necessary because airlines don't carry many extra meals (if any at all) on their aircraft just in case. In fact they would have to stock a bewildering combination if they did. The big airlines have a whole host of special meals, including simple vegetarian, and those for medical-based diets (e.g. gluten-free or diabetic) and for religious diets (e.g. kosher and halal). Some airlines will provide all meals in a special form – for example, Malaysian Airlines' food is all halal.

→ Fast Track: Special Meal Types

Exact meal specifications vary from airline to airline, but these are a common selection. The meal codes are set by the international IATA organization.

Medical	
Meal	*Code*
Diabetic	DBML
Gluten-free	GFML
Low-sodium (low-salt)	LSML
Low-cholesterol	LFML
Low-calorie	LCML
Low-protein potassium	LPML
High-fibre	HFML
Bland (low-residue/gastric)	BLML
Low-purine (uric acid)	PRML
Non-lactose	NLML
Special medical requirements	SPML*

Vegetarian

Meal	Code
Lacto-ovo vegetarian	VLML
Vegan (non-dairy)	VGML
Asian vegetarian	AVML

Religious

Meal	Code
Hindu	HNML
Kosher	KSML
Muslim	MOML

Children's

Meal	Code
Child	CHML
Baby	BBML

Other

Meal	Code
Seafood	SFML
Fruit plate	FPML

* This is not a standard IATA code, but is used by some airlines to denote a one-off special meal for other medical requirements.

Just because you ask for a 'special' meal doesn't make it any better than the usual fare. Although there has been some improvement, many airlines' vegetarian selections are frankly boring. You may also face incomprehension on the part of the cabin crew, as my vegan colleague (see page 186) found out to his cost.

✈ *Summary:* The Special-Needs Traveller

- Let the airline know at reservation of any special needs you may have.

- Reconfirm your special needs at check-in.

- Allow extra time if you have a wheelchair or other equipment to be dealt with.

- If you want to take your wheelchair into the cabin, get in early. Not all aircraft have space, and the cabin will not accommodate all wheelchairs.

- If your chair has wet-cell batteries it will not be allowed in the cabin and will take extra time to pack in the hold.

- Oxygen can be supplied if requested (at a fee), but you can't take your own oxygen bottles on board.

- Guide dogs and other helping animals can usually travel with you for free.

- Check if your condition requires a medical certificate.

- Cabin crew are limited in the assistance they are allowed to give. Check that you will not need a carer to accompany you.

- As with all other special-needs requirements, the airline will need advance warning to supply special meals.

13 Sky Pets

Travelling with pets can be even harder than travelling with children. You don't have to keep the pet entertained on board, and you won't have to change any nappies in difficult conditions, but the paperwork is more complicated and you have to make absolutely sure beforehand that you have done everything to make your pet's journey comfortable.

Transporting animals

The pet transport plan begins with a suitable carrier. It is not enough to pop your pet in a cardboard box. It needs to be in a rigid carrier with plenty of air holes and enough space for it to be able to lie down comfortably away from any droppings and to be able to turn round.

On top of this you will need to supply sufficient food and water to keep your pet happy. But this can't be just popped in a bowl at the bottom of the carrier, as the water will soon be splashed all over. You will need to invest in an appropriate water dispenser.

Get your pet used to the carrier well before the journey. Have it open in the house, and let your pet wander in and out of it. You may like to move your pet's bedding into the carrier, again leaving the door open.

When the day to travel comes, have a supply of titbits and small toys to keep your pet occupied. Put some comfortable bedding in the carrier. Maximize contact when you are able to do so. Try to make the journey minimally painful for your pet.

Quick Tip: **Pets are Excess Baggage . . . except Guide Dogs**

Pets are generally treated as excess baggage, even if you could fit them within your baggage limits, so you have to pay for their transport. One exception is guide dogs, which are usually allowed to fly for free in addition to the normal free baggage allowance.

Cabin or hold?

Larger animals will have to travel in the hold, but a pet whose travelling case can fit under the seat in front of you will often be allowed on board. This tends to restrict the availability to cats and smaller dogs (guide dogs and guide monkeys get special treatment in this respect).

If it is possible for your pet to travel in the cabin it will probably find the experience more pleasant than going in the hold – ask at reservation whether or not it is possible. You should still take up all the above suggestions for what to include with the pet carrier, though. Assume that your pet is going to spend the entire time in the carrier, and stock up accordingly. There may be some problem when you arrive at the airport that means it has to travel in the hold after all, and even in the cabin it may spend a fair amount of time in the carrier. Take with you appropriate materials to clear up any mess it might make – the crew are not going to respond kindly to requests to deal with dog poo.

Don't panic if your pet has to fly in the hold. It is a perfectly acceptable environment – it will be lit and heated, and have air at the same pressure as in the cabin.

Medical care

Animals find the experience of air travel stressful. Even if you manage to get your pet in the cabin with you, it is a strange environment with unfamiliar sounds, sights and smells. If the animal has to travel in the hold, it is going to be bundled up in a travelling carrier potentially for many hours and moved around, perhaps with slightly less care and attention than you normally give it.

At one time it was common practice to sedate pets for travel, but an unacceptable number died in transit as a result of the sedation and the practice is no longer recommended. It is a good idea to consult your vet before travel, to check if there are any special needs your pet might have.

Pet paperwork

Until recently, UK-based cat and dog owners and those travelling into the UK were faced with a terrible choice. Either their animal was left behind or they faced an expensive six-month quarantine period. The reason for these extreme measures was the very effective campaign to keep rabies off the island.

Now things are much better. The pet-passport scheme, which was launched in February 2000, means that it is possible to bring a suitably certified cat or dog into the country from twenty-two other European countries without any quarantine. In 2001 the scheme was extended to include a range of long-haul destinations, including Australia, Japan, New Zealand and Singapore along with much of the West Indies. However, it still does not include the USA and Canada.

This scheme – known as PETS (PEt Travel Scheme) – does not mean, however, that the process is either quick or cheap. To be able to use the scheme, your pet will need to be microchipped for positive identification, will need a suitable pet passport, and will need to have a vet's certificate establishing that it has been vaccinated against rabies and is rabies-free.

→ **Fast Track:
Pet Passports**

*For a cat or dog to enter the UK from an appropriate European
country on a pet passport it has to*

* be implanted with a microchip to give it a unique identity
  number;

* be vaccinated against rabies;

* have a blood test a month later to ensure the vaccine is
  effective;

* have a second blood test six months later before the pet can
  come back to the UK;

* get a PETS certificate.

Also,

* the day before arriving back in port, it must be treated for
  tapeworm and ticks by a registered vet;

* the animal must be brought in on an authorized PETS route;

* you must sign a declaration of residency to say that the animal
  hasn't been outside an authorized country.

For a long-haul country your pet also has to

* travel in a container with a seal that shows that it has not
  been opened en route;

* have an import licence;

* comply with any special requirements for individual countries.

Some pet owners fight shy of PETS because they don't like the sound of having their dog or cat microchipped. In fact this is a valuable safeguard for any pet, irrespective of whether it is going to fly. If your animal gets loose and is picked up, any vet or animal-welfare organization and many police stations will be able to scan for a chip, find the animal's registration number, and use it look up your pet in a centrally held database, where it is registered for life.

We recently had a dog microchipped, and the experience was no more difficult for the animal than having an inoculation. The chip is tiny – about the size of a grain of rice – and is sealed in a glass cylinder. It is injected under the skin of the animal, usually in the loose skin around the neck. There are no marks, nor is there any lump you can feel. When your dog or cat has to be scanned, a simple hand scanner is passed over it – it's a very simple, painless process. In the early days of chipping there was some confusion caused by incompatible standards of chips and readers, but there is now an international standard – make sure the chip you have implanted is compatible with ISO 11784/5.

The UK Department for Environment, Food and Rural Affairs web site (see page 327) has up-to-date information on PETS. The intention is to extend the scheme to other potential rabies carriers currently requiring quarantine. These include chinchillas, gerbils, guinea pigs, hamsters, mice, rabbits and rats. This list isn't exhaustive – check before deciding to import an animal.

Other animals still need appropriate import documentation, and this is true of most countries around the world. Rabies-susceptible animals from other countries will also have to pass through the quarantine procedure. It is up to you to pay for the quarantine. The DEFRA site gives details of quarantine facilities. You will also have to obtain an import licence – again there is information on the Ministry site, and the quarantine location will usually obtain the licence for you.

The UK is not the only country or island to enforce quarantine, and not everywhere has yet adopted a similar pet-passport scheme. For instance, Hawaii insists on quarantining animals, as it is in a similar position to the UK in being an island off a rabies-infected mainland. Check the DEFRA web site (see page 327) for more information on the requirements for taking your pet to a particular country.

✈ *Summary:* Sky Pets

- Use appropriate travelling cases that are both strong and spacious enough for your animals.

- Think through the animal's journey, and make sure that all its requirements have been catered for.

- Take your animal in the cabin if possible.

- Take your vet's advice, but be wary of sedation.

- Make sure that you plan the appropriate pet paperwork well in advance.

- Be prepared for expensive and lengthy quarantine when entering some countries if there is no pet-passport scheme.

14 Complaints Please!

With the best will in the world, air travel will sometimes go wrong. The less customer-aware airlines and travel companies can be extremely slippery when it comes to compensation. This chapter is a guide to getting things fixed when they go awry.

Motivate to assist

If the problem arises part-way through your journey, your biggest friend will be an ability to keep calm. This doesn't mean that you have to be a doormat, giving way to every whim and suggestion of the airline. However, storming up to the airline's desk and yelling at the poor representative while slamming your fist on the counter will rarely get the best result. In fact many agents delight in making things tough for their 'difficult' customers.

You are much more likely to get positive action by motivating the airline staff to help you. Sympathize with them. Say that you understand their problems, and that you understand that it isn't their fault personally. And then ask, 'But isn't there something you could do to help?' Make your requests practicable. There is no point asking for a replacement aircraft if yours has gone missing, but you can ask for your wait to be minimized and made as comfortable as possible.

You may find that there is some benefit in making use of the other passengers to emulate the classic interrogation technique of alternating nasty and nice questioners. Wait until an agent has been verbally assaulted by a particularly unpleasant passenger, then go up, sympathize, agree what a pain people like 'him' are (immediately making you and the agent into 'us'), and then make your specific, practical request.

→ Fast Track: Motivation Mnemonic

It can help to keep some key points in mind when trying to get your own way. Try staying SHARP:

- *S – Sympathize –* get on the agents' side, understand how difficult it is for them, but . . .

- *H – Help –* ask for help. Don't demand: try to get them in a position where they feel that they need to defend you. This may require you to be . . .

- *A – Assertive –* sometimes you will have to ask for what you need over and over. Never get aggressive, always be pleasant, but keep pressing your point. You can make this more attractive to the agents by using . . .

- *R – Reward* – the more they can get out of helping you, the more they will want to help. It all starts with frequent 'thank you' smiles and eye contact – one of the simplest but best rewards. If they're good, tell them they're good. But, however well they are rewarded, you will need to be . . .

- *P – Practicable* – there is no point asking for a new aircraft or crew to be materialized out of thin air. Stretch what is offered, but think through what is practicable.

Bags on the run

Baggage goes adrift remarkably often. As many as one in twelve passengers who put bags in the hold lose something. A fair amount of this lost luggage is not so much lost as misdirected, ending up at the wrong destination without you. It may well find its way home with a little help from the airline. In fact 98 per cent of lost bags do turn up. But, given the number of bags in the system, that still leaves plenty going missing – and more that turn up in a damaged state. To make matters worse, the airlines have unusually strong protection against financial claims, thanks to the Warsaw Convention (see below), their safety blanket dating back to the earliest days of air travel.

The Warsaw Convention is a handy piece of inter-national legislation that limits the airline's responsibility. Hardly any other industry is so cushioned from the effects of mistreating its customers. The international limits of liability are around $20 per kilogram (with a $400 limit

Quick Tip: Keep It to Hand

The simplest way to keep your luggage and valuables safe is to make sure that you don't hand them over to anyone else and don't let them be put in the hold. With the best will in the world, baggage handlers are going to throw bags around. I've loaded aircraft in my time, and it is physically impossible to get bags into some of the places you have to without throwing them. So limit yourself to hand baggage that can be carried on the plane and you will minimize the risk.

on unchecked baggage) up to the maximum the airline allows for checked baggage – usually meaning a maximum of $640 per bag. In the huge US internal market there used to be a limit of $1,250, but this has gone up to $2,500.

That doesn't cover all your goods either. You can wave goodbye to any currency, high-value electronics and precious goods like jewellery and paintings, unless you have made special arrangements with the airline or an insurer. (Some credit-card companies provide this sort of cover if your air tickets are bought with the card.) You won't get a new-for-old replacement from an airline as you would with an ordinary insurance claim either – the airline is able to apply depreciation to the value of your goods. It isn't fair, but there is no point blustering: the airlines have the force of law behind them. If you want a hobby, feel free to campaign for a change to international law, but otherwise it's best to accept the situation with good grace.

What about claiming compensation for any damage that *you* might suffer, say from bad air? Again the Warsaw Convention takes the stage. Back in 1929, when this international agreement was signed, governments were more closely tied into the airline business. Many airlines were 'national carriers', an extension of the government. As crashes were relatively common then, the governments put the main burden on the passenger, a deadly caveat emptor that said that the passenger, by flying, accepted the risk of the activity. It is a bit like one of those disclaimers you sign when you go bungee jumping or white-water rafting.

Now, when air travel is a commonplace, it is bizarre that this extreme-risk approach exists to cap any claims for compensation, but the Warsaw Convention remains in force. Effectively, airlines are above the law – figuratively as well as literally.

→ Fast Track:
The Warsaw Convention

The Warsaw Convention originated in 1929 and covers airlines' international liability. Over 120 countries are signatories.

• The original liability limits were specified in terms of the French franc 'consisting of 65 mg of gold'. In 1929 the 125,000-franc personal-liability limit was thought to be worth around $100,000, but it is not clear if the limit is based on exchange rate or gold value. There is no allowance for inflation built into the Convention.

- Airline implementations of the Convention usually state liability in terms of SDR (special drawing rights). These are units used by the International Monetary Fund. At the time of writing, 1 SDR is worth $1.27 or 88p.

- Personal liability is limited to 50,000 SDR if there was no 'wilful misconduct' on the part of the airline ($63,500 or £44,000 at the time of writing).

- The major airlines also subscribe to a 1990s IATA (International Air Transport Association) agreement whereby airlines agree to accept liability for claims up to 100,000 SDR ($127,000 or £88,000 at the time of writing) without resorting to legal defence and to have no cap if families can prove damages beyond this.

- Baggage-loss liability is limited to 17 SDR ($21.59 or £14.96 at the time of writing) per kilogram, with a limit of 332 SDR ($421.64 or £292.16 at the time of writing) on unchecked baggage. If your checked-baggage weight is not recorded it is assumed to be the free limit.

- If passengers are not issued with a ticket stating the place and date of issue, the place of departure, the destination, and that travel is subject to the Convention, the airline will not be able to make use of the provisions of the Convention.

- The Warsaw Convention does not specify compensatory damage for families of passengers killed in an air crash.

- The Warsaw Convention requires that a claim be made within two years from the date on which the aircraft should have arrived. However, many airlines limit damage-claim notification to seven days and delayed-baggage claims to twenty-one days.

- Under the Warsaw Convention, lawsuits can be filed in one
  of four possible places, or 'venues': (1) the country where
  the passenger purchased the ticket, (2) the country of the
  passenger's final destination, (3) the country where the airline
  is incorporated, or (4) the country where the airline maintains
  its principal place of business.

The empty carousel

We have all been in arrival halls and waited for what
seemed like hours for our bags to appear on the carousel.
But what should you do when a bag doesn't turn up? Make
sure all the bags are through. If they are, and yours is
missing, don't leave the airport without acceptance of this
in writing from the airline, otherwise it can be difficult to
prove anything after the event. Make sure you are given a
contact number for chasing up progress.

So now you are in what could be a strange location
without essential baggage. First, make sure that you are
going to get the missing bags delivered to wherever you are
staying without extra cost. As usual, there's no obligation
on the airline, but it will normally provide this service.
Then see if there is any way it can help out. Airlines
normally carry emergency kits if you have lost the basics
(though they may well limit these to international customers). They can also provide you with some expenses.
Surprise, surprise – they have no obligation to do so.

Demanding will get you nowhere. Be friendly and
understanding, but be assertive. Agree with the agent, be

sympathetic, but keep coming back to what you want. 'I understand – it's a pain for you. But you can see how it is. Without my bags I am going to have buy a new shirt for the presentation I have to give this afternoon. What do you think is a reasonable amount to buy one here?' The amount given is usually at the discretion of the person on the desk. Again, use charm not aggression. If you try to go over his or her head by demanding to see the supervisor, the agent will be backed up to the hilt. Don't threaten – encourage.

Once you are past your immediate requirement, if your bags are still missing make sure that you fill in an appropriate form in time. There is usually a time limit in which claims must be put in – often a week. Bearing in mind that handling your claim requires good communication between the customer-contact staff at the airport and the back-office people handling claims, it is a good idea if you take charge of this process and make sure you get the claim in, rather than assuming that they will make it all happen.

✔ Checklist: Preparing for a Baggage Claim

- ❑ Use charm, not aggression.
- ❑ Insist that the attendant fills out a missing-baggage report, even if you are assured that the bags are coming on the next flight.
- ❑ Fill in the form on the spot.
- ❑ Take a copy of the missing-baggage report with you, even if you are assured that everything will be handled for you.

❑ Get names and contact details of the staff involved.

❑ Get the airline's policies on free delivery, reimbursement, acceptable delay etc. in writing.

❑ Establish any time limit on claims.

❑ If you have a camera with you, take photographs of damaged baggage immediately after you receive it.

❑ Keep all damaged baggage, including locks, broken security bands etc.

❑ Include copies of all supporting documents with your claim.

Delays, delays

As a source of frustration, lost bags are almost equalled by the news that your plane has been delayed. It's going to happen occasionally even in the best-run airline. Commercial airliners are incredibly expensive – we are dealing with billion-dollar vehicles – and airlines can't afford to keep stacks of planes on standby, just in case one goes wrong. The really big airlines might have a few fallback aircraft at their main centres of operation, but that's about it. So when an aircraft goes wrong there will be delays – and not just to the immediate flight, as there will be knock-on effects for later flights in the day. It is probably worth asking yourself if you would rather they made certain the plane was safe to fly, or took a risk with your life.

Rather more delays come from outside sources – from air traffic control and weather and the myriad problems that can influence the complex dance that is a plane journey.

Again, there is little point in getting too stroppy with the airline representative because the delay has happened. And also again, the Warsaw Convention is quite clear that you have no rights – there is no compensation requirement for flight delays, however long they may be.

Even more so than with missing bags, you are going to control how much help the airline will give you by the way you react. If you can be positive but assertive you will get much further than either the aggressive angry person or the doormat that simply follows instructions. You should expect attempts to get you on another flight – potentially with another airline – or to provide something to eat and if necessary a hotel room. But don't act as if this is a God-given right. You will get the best results from charm.

Feeling the bump

We are developing a compensation culture. When something goes wrong, the first thing we want to do is find someone to blame. Then we look for redress. We want to have things made better. Airlines are better protected than most against the need to compensate. As we have seen, there is no requirement for the airlines to provide you with compensation if you are delayed or your flight is cancelled. The only real legal certainty is that you are owed some compensation if you are 'bumped' – the flight is overbooked and you are prevented from flying involuntarily. Then most countries require their airlines to take action.

In the vast majority of cases, however, there will be no compensation. Certainly don't look for any recompense for any loss of business you may experience as a result of missing a flight. The airline has no interest in the fact that you missed closing a deal or giving a seminar, or couldn't get to your granny's ninetieth-birthday party.

→ Fast Track: Your Limited Rights

Thanks to the web of legislation that the Warsaw Convention weaves around air flight, your rights are strictly limited.

Problem	Rights
Delayed baggage	No rights at all. Discretionary 'emergency' kits and payments. Discretionary delivery of baggage to your final destination
Lost or damaged weighed baggage	Up to approximately £14.96 (see page 250 on SDR values) per kilogram, depending on the depreciated value of the contents
Lost or damaged unweighed baggage	Up to approximately £14.96 (see page 250 on SDR values) times your baggage allowance in kilograms, depending on the depreciated value of the contents
Delays and cancellations	You should be carried on a later flight at no extra charge. No compensation. Accommodation and meals at airline's discretion

Voluntary 'bumping'	Whatever is agreed between you and the airline
Involuntary 'bumping'	No compensation for lost business etc. USA – nothing for under an hour's delay, one-way fare up to $200 for up to two hours' delay, twice one-way fare up to $400 for over two hours UK – airline's discretion. BA operates £150 short-haul, £200 long-haul.
Injury and death	Personal liability cover up to around £44,000 (see page 250 on SDR values), but up to £88,000 unlikely to be contested

Getting your own back

If you can't sort things out at the airport, you may still want to see if you can get something out of the airline for your trouble. There are a few simple tips that will help maximize your chances of being successful in this.

Begin by making notes (or use a voice recorder) on the spot. Get the name of any airline representatives involved in the problem. Keep a note of times and locations. Keep all the documents that refer to your travel, as well as receipts for any expenses you incur as a result of the problem. Before you leave the airport, find out the address of the airline's corporate headquarters or customer-service department.

When you then contact the airline, it is best to do so in writing with a signed letter rather than using an e-mail, which is still regarded as less significant by many businesses. Keep the letter short – down to a single page if you can. Highlight the key points – think of your letter as a sales pitch in which you don't want the recipient to get bored or lose track part-way through. Attach photocopies of any documentation that backs up your claim, but not the originals. And make sure that you give daytime contact details, so that the airline can carry the investigation forward.

Keep the letter as businesslike as possible. Any tendency to sink into abuse will mean that it will get disregarded as ranting. Be practical and realistic. When mentioning employees, name both those who were rude and made things worse and those who were helpful – there's nothing wrong with including praise in a letter of complaint. Most important of all, keep the letter focused on the problem in hand and the action you want the airline to take. Don't let it drift off into your favourite topics and bugbears.

→ Fast Track: Making a Complaint

- Make notes (or record them) on the spot.

- Get the names of any airline staff involved.

- Note times and locations.

- Keep all documents (e.g. baggage stubs).

- Find out the address of the airline's corporate headquarters and customer-service department.

- Contact the airline in writing.

- Keep the letter down to a single page.

- Attach copies of all documentation.

- Mention both negative and positive points and staff.

- Stick to the point.

- Give your daytime contact details.

Some countries have bodies that are specifically intended to help passengers who are having trouble with airlines. In the UK, the consumer watchdog is the Air Transport Users Council (0207 240 6061, see page 326 for its web site). You can also complain about an airline to the body that deals with civil aviation in the appropriate country – the Civil Aviation Authority in the UK, the Department of Transportation in the US – but don't expect a quick response or any action specific to your case. You may influence future guidelines and laws, but probably won't get any personal benefit.

✈ *Summary:* **Complaints Please!**

- Keep calm.

- Get the airline employees to help – don't put their backs up.

- Stick to hand baggage if you can.

- Be aware of the limits imposed by the Warsaw Convention.

- Be systematic when making a complaint.

- Be aware of your rights – and where the airline employee might have some leeway.

- Use a letter rather than the phone or e-mail to complain after the event.

15 How Safe is Safe?
A Guide to Staying Airborne

Air travel is very safe – as the airlines never tire of telling us. However, airline companies have, by mutual agreement, never competed on safety, nor will you ever find 'safety' mentioned in any airline advertisement. Safety is, quite simply, not a competitive issue. But for us, the passengers, it has supreme importance.

An airliner is not a natural environment. As any airline pilot will tell you, a jet aircraft has all the gliding capability of a brick. It's only superb design, maintenance, flight-crew capability and air traffic control that keep us alive. This chapter explores the realities of survival. The airlines are fond of telling us that it is safer to fly than to travel by road, but what does this mean? Just what do the statistics comparing flight with other forms of travel actually tell us? What are the realities of airline safety?

Flying by numbers

Understanding what the safety statistics mean is not just a matter of idle curiosity. It can help nervous fliers put their fear into perspective. But there is a problem. The statistics of survival are about probabilities, and there is something in the human brain that seems designed to reject the reality of probability. At first glance, probabilities bear no good relationship to common sense. You have only to look at the immense profits made by casinos and the betting industry to see that our natural grasp of probability is weak.

If you are not comfortable with the basics of probability, the airline safety statistics will be of no value. For this reason I am going to spend a few paragraphs removing the obscurity from probability first. If you are happy with the workings of probability, or just can't be bothered, skip over the Fast Track section below. But be warned: without overcoming your natural reaction to probability you won't be able to make sense of the statistics.

→ Fast Track:
Taking Chances

Probability is the science of chance, and lies at the heart of all the airline statistics and comparisons with other forms of transport. Most airline statistics involve very large numbers, but to keep the explanations simple I am going to stick to a familiar vehicle of probability that requires only small numbers – a dice.

Dice have six sides and throwing one produces a random selection from the six numbers it carries, so we say that there's a 1 in 6 chance of getting a particular throw. Let's say I throw a three, then throw the dice again. Here's where common sense goes out of the window. It seems natural to assume that there is less chance of getting a three this time. In fact, though, the dice has no memory. Once again there is exactly a 1 in 6 chance of getting any particular throw.

So doesn't this mean that I could throw three after three after three – say ten times over? Yes it does. But it is very unlikely. There are millions of different combinations of those ten dice throws. Each individual combination has exactly the same chance of occurring – but all but one will not produce a three for each throw. Because of this low chance of getting ten sequential threes, it seems particularly unlikely that the final throw will also come up three if we've already got a three for each of the last nine throws. But, as we have already seen, the dice has no memory. At this point there is still a 1 in 6 chance that the result will be three.

On average, over time, there will be the same number of ones, twos, threes, fours, fives and sixes thrown – but it can take a long time for things to even out.

The other thing that it's important to understand is the way in which probabilities add together. If there is a 1 in 6 chance of getting a three when you throw one dice, what is the chance of getting a three on either of two dice? This is important because, thinking of accident statistics, we need to know not just the chance of a crash if we take one flight, but the chance of a crash on any of the flights we are taking.

It would be simple if we could just add the probabilities together. There is a 1 in 6 chance on the first dice and a 1 in 6 chance on the second, so could the chance of getting a three on either of the dice be 1 + 1, i.e. 2 in 6? Unfortunately it isn't that simple, otherwise by throwing a dice six times you could guarantee that you would get a three. Real life doesn't work that way.

Mathematicians have come up with a method of combining probabilities, though. The reasoning is obscure, but the result is quite simple. If there is a 1 in 6 chance of getting a three, that means there is a 5 in 6 chance of not getting a three. To combine a pair of 5 in 6 chances of not getting threes, they are multiplied together, so that there is therefore a 25 in 36 chance of not getting a three from either of two dice. That means an 11 in 36 chance that you *will* get a three on one of the two dice. Note that this is slightly less than the 12 in 36 (2 in 6) chance we would have got by adding the probabilities together. This slight reduction ensures that, though it gets more and more likely that we will get a three as we throw many times, it is never certain.

With these two facts firmly established – that probability has no memory and so is not influenced by past results, and that probabilities combine in this rather odd reversed multiplication – we can return to the realities of surviving a crash.

Is flying safer than driving?

Let's look at those statistics. Probably the best comparison for the safety of flying is with the car, a means of transport most of us don't think twice before using. The trouble is, the comparison can be misleading. Take media coverage. Plane crashes are dramatic and relatively rare, so they inevitably make headline news. Car crashes happen every day. There are around 100 people involved in fatal or serious accidents each day in the UK alone. This makes the 'ordinary' car accident not worthy of news attention, however distressing it is for those involved, so we get a totally artificial picture of the dangers of air travel from the news.

Equally misleading, but in a different way, is the comparison of outcomes. There are a few hundred people killed worldwide in plane crashes each year. By comparison, more than 40,000 people die annually in car crashes in the USA alone. But this misses an obvious difference. Most of us take many more car trips than air flights, so it's not enough to say that flying is safer than car travel just because many fewer people are killed that way each year.

The two types of journey are sometimes compared on distance – how safe they are per kilometre travelled – but again this comparison is almost meaningless. What we really want to know is, 'What is the chance that something nasty is going to happen to *me* on *this* flight (the one I'm about to take) and how does it compare with the chance of something nasty happening to *me* on *that* car journey?'

On average, fatal aircraft accidents occur in 1 in 1 million flights. Literally 1 in 1 million. Not odds that many would bother with when betting. Things are even better when you consider UK-registered aircraft, which did not have a single fatal accident between 1900 and 1999, despite clocking up 7.5 million take-offs and landings. You can see more specific figures for different airlines on page 310, but the average is better than 1 in 1 million.

By comparison, in the UK the chances of being killed in a car accident in one year is about 6 in 100,000 for adults. The statistics here aren't quite comparable, though. We make an average of 650 car journeys each per year. By plugging in the numbers, this makes the chances of being in a fatal accident on any one journey around 1 in 10 million – a little better than a single plane journey. On the other hand, if you'd like to make the comparison the other way around, an average traveller may take ten air flights in a year – that makes the chances of being in a crash in that year rather better than 1 in 100,000, against the 6 in 100,000 on the road.

Quick Tip: **Fly Non-Stop**

There's a simple but satisfying way to decrease the risk of a crash on your journey. As most fatal accidents occur during take-off, climb, descent and landing (despite popular opinion, the worst time is climb, followed by landing), you can instantly reduce the risk you are exposed to by reducing the number of take-offs and landings. Going for a non-stop flight is a no-brainer.

If the car journey appears safer than you might imagine, remember that we're talking fatal accidents in these statistics. Plane crashes are much more likely to involve fatalities than car crashes. I've personally been in at least five car accidents already. There are 100 times as many people with reported injuries in car accidents than are killed, and many more unreported accidents, or accidents that don't involve injury. You are *much* more likely to have an accident on a car journey than on a flight – but the comparison of fatal accidents gives a more effective perspective.

Let's put that annual chance of being in a fatal plane crash up against an extremely unlikely risk. The chances of being killed by a lightning strike during a single year in the UK is around 10 million to 1. By comparison, the chances of being killed on a flight is about 8 million to 1 worldwide – a very similar risk. But few of us refuse ever to go outside just in case lightning strikes. Admittedly the lightning statistic is for the whole year, while the chance of dying in a plane crash is for a single flight, but even so it puts the risk into context.

The fact is, the statistics are encouraging. They will rarely be enough alone to overcome fear (see page 160) – after all, that fear is a natural survival reaction. But the numbers can help bring a degree of rationality back into the way we look at air travel.

A safer airline

One other use of the statistics, apart from getting an overall feel for just how safe it is to fly, is to compare different airlines. The tables in Appendix 3 show how different airlines have fared over a thirty-year period. There is some variation, but it would be unrealistic to say that it proves anything in most cases. Because we are dealing with a small number of incidents in the overall operations, just one accident makes the difference between a 'perfect' record and a less encouraging one.

Mathematicians would say that the differences between many airlines are not 'statistically significant'. The point is, if you throw a coin four times, on average you are going to get two heads and two tails. But it doesn't mean that there's anything wrong with the coin if you get three heads and one tail. It's not statistically significant – there hasn't been enough opportunity for everything to even itself out. The same is true with the small numbers of accidents that most airlines have suffered.

A study of major US airlines by Arnold Barnett and Alexander Wang (*Flight Safety Digest*, April 2000) looked back over a ten-year period from 1996. During that time, USAir (now US Airways) had the worst record, with a probability of an individual being killed on one of its flights of 1 in 2.5 million. This compared with other airlines with rates as low as 1 in 53 million, and some with no accidents at all. But, for the numbers involved, these differences were not significant – there was no evidence that USAir was any worse than the rest. The authors point out that the airline's performance, while five times worse than the collective result in that period, was five times better in the previous ten years, emphasizing the random nature of the result when long-term fluctuations are taken into account.

Only those airlines with an extreme record really need consideration. From the data in Appendix 3 (page 310) it seems that, looking at the whole world's airlines over a longer period, there are a handful which have sufficiently high scores to suggest that there may be some point in avoiding their flights.

It is unfortunate that the records for the airlines of the

former Soviet Union are so chaotic that there can't be a proper comparison made, as there is a significant suspicion that there may be extra problems attached to these airlines. From the little data that is available, you will see that the statistics for these airlines stand out as particularly worrying. But it is clear that the decision is not as simple as 'stick to US airlines' or 'stick to European airlines' for a safer flight.

A safer route

The Barnett and Wang study went on to compare US airlines with other 'advanced-world' carriers (defined as being in 'economically advanced, technologically advanced and politically democratic countries') and 'developing-world' carriers. This part of the study had particularly interesting results. The first was to show that the US carriers were no safer than their advanced-world equivalents. In fact the results showed a rather worse fatality rate for US carriers (though, again, not big enough to be statistically meaningful). This runs totally counter to the impression (particularly prevalent in the USA) that US airlines are the safest in the world.

Most fascinating of all was the comparison with the 'developing-world' airlines. With these the risk was around ten times as high – a big enough difference to imply that there was a real trend in place. The knee-jerk reaction would be to say, 'Let's avoid the airlines from the developing world.' Only it's not that simple. If you compare the performance of developing-world airlines and advanced-world airlines on the same routes there is no real difference. The fact is that there is a higher risk when flying on routes between advanced-world countries and developing-world countries, or between developing-world countries, than there is when flying between advanced-world countries. As developing-world airlines fly a higher percentage of these high-risk routes, they will have a worse record.

Why should these routes cause problems? Because the causes of an aircraft accident are not limited to the airline. There can be involvement from air traffic control, from the airport, and from the local ground maintenance. It seems that, for the most part, if you need to go to one of the higher-risk destinations it doesn't matter from a safety standpoint which airline you choose. But even there we are talking about a risk of being killed of no worse than 600,000 to 1 against – not exactly a gambler's certainty.

Plane preferences

Perhaps more significant than the airlines' records are those of the planes, as there are fewer different models, and, while most airlines strive for safety, it is quite possible for some airliners to be less safe than others. The tables in Appendix 4 give a picture of the performance of the most common Western jets. Unfortunately, appropriate data is not available for the airlines and planes of the former Soviet Union. This is a shame, as there is some subjective evidence that these airlines and particularly these aircraft have not got a safety record comparable to those of their counterparts in the rest of the world.

Quick Tip: Think Big

Aircraft that carry thirty or more passengers are subject to significantly more stringent safety checks and maintenance than smaller planes. Small aircraft are statistically more risky to fly in, and are more likely to result in total fatality if there should be a serious accident.

It might seem that one obvious factor in plane reliability is age. We know that our cars typically get less reliable as they get older. But this reflects how cars are built and maintained rather than anything more definitive. Although there is an increased risk of metal fatigue as an airframe gets older, the maintenance an aircraft undergoes is so rigorous that any parts liable to introduce danger are replaced before there is a serious risk.

Once an aircraft has got over any technical teething troubles of newness it usually remains at a fairly constant level of safety, unless maintenance measures are not adequate. Again, due to lack of detailed information, there has to be some doubt about the level of maintenance on some aircraft of the former Soviet Union, so it is arguable that if any type of plane should be avoided it is an ageing ex-Eastern Bloc jet.

Belt up

It is quite amazing how a ripple of clunks goes around the cabin the moment the captain switches off the 'Fasten seat belts' sign. By all means loosen your belt a little, but it's worth leaving it fastened at all times when you have no good reason to be unstrapped. Clear-air turbulence, which can make the plane drop several thousand feet with no warning, does happen. The result has been head injuries as passengers fly into the air and collide with the overhead lockers and the ceiling, or when they fall back to the floor.

There is no requirement to unfasten your seat belt – so why do it? In non-fatal accidents, turbulence is the biggest cause of injuries to both passengers and crew. Each year in the USA alone over fifty passengers are injured by turbulence while not wearing their seat belts. Of the three passengers killed and eighty seriously injured due to turbulence in US flights between 1981 and 1997, 'at least' two of the three killed and seventy-three of those seriously injured weren't wearing seat belts.

Medical emergencies

We have seen the message of the statistics, but there is one other survivability factor that differs from airline to airline. If you develop a serious medical condition on board you will be dependent on whatever facilities the aircraft carries. At the time of writing, only a small number of airlines include more than a basic medical kit. A few, like American Airlines, British Airways, Lufthansa and Swissair, carry defibrillators – essential to maximize the chance of surviving a heart stoppage.

The airline should be able to tell you at the time of booking whether or not it is company policy to carry defibrillators, though they will not be able to guarantee whether or not one will be carried on your flight.

While it may be of no particular value to your own safety, you may like to consider taking a basic first-aid course and brushing up on the essentials of resuscitation in case you are on a flight where someone is taken ill. However, unless you are medically trained, the cabin crew are liable to have an equivalent or better level of first-aid knowledge.

✈ *Summary:* How Safe is Safe

- Probability has no memory – the chance of a crash happening on one flight is not influenced by how many previous safe flights you have had.

- The chance of a fatal accident happening on a particular flight is around 1 in 1 million – compared with the chance of a fatal accident on a particular car journey of around 1 in 10 million . . .

- . . . but we take more car journeys in a year, so for someone taking ten flights a year the chance of being involved in a fatal plane crash is rather better than 1 in 100,000, versus 6 in 100,000 on the road.

- Flying non-stop reduces take-offs and landings, the most dangerous part of flight.

- Excluding ex-Soviet Union airlines, no airlines stand out as particularly dangerous, but routes to and from the developing world *are* more dangerous.

- Large aircraft (those carrying more than thirty passengers) tend to be significantly safer than smaller planes.

- Some aircraft seem to be slightly safer than others – best avoided are ageing ex-Eastern Bloc aircraft.

- Keeping your seat belt fastened throughout the flight reduces the risk of turbulence injury.

16 Crash Landing – Surviving the Unthinkable

First the good news. Every month there are hundreds of minor aircraft problems that seem life-threatening at the time to the passengers, but prove harmless. Airlines' incident reports can sound dramatic. To the passengers on board an aircraft when 'there was a loud bang and the port engine ran down [i.e. stopped]' or 'the landing gear failed to lock in place despite repeated attempts' it might have seemed that a crash was imminent, but the final result was a safe landing with no injuries. As we have seen, the chance of a fatal accident occurring is literally one in a million chance.

However, crashes and accidents *do* happen, and then it's up to the passenger to manage his or her own survival. In fact your chances are getting better all the time. The survival rate for air crashes is now well over 50 per cent – twice what it was a couple of decades ago.

First steps to survival

Your first chance to enhance your ability to survive has already passed once you've accepted a seat. By going for an aisle seat near an emergency exit you reduce the journey you have to make from your seat to get out of the plane. Remember, after a crash the cabin will be in confusion (see Jerry Schemmel's graphic account on page 281). You will be disoriented. If there isn't immediately, there will probably soon be smoke inside the cabin. You want to make it as simple as you can to get to the exits.

Some experts suggest going for seats in the mid-section of the plane, near the wings. There is some evidence that there's a slightly higher chance of surviving in this area. If there is a better chance, it is probably because the airframe there is strengthened to cope with the stresses put on it by the wings. However, it is also true that the sides of the aircraft there may be more liable to damage if the wings are ripped off.

Something else you can do just in case is to get the route to the emergency exits firmly in mind. Count the numbers of rows of seats between you and the nearest exits. Look for exits both ways. In some crashes, passengers have died when the obvious exit was blocked, but they could have gone the other way to safety.

Wear sensible clothes, too. Anything highly flammable is an obvious choice to avoid. Shorts, short skirts and skimpy shirts won't give you the protection you need. For footwear, stay away from anything sharp. It is also sensible to check that you don't have items about your person that could do you an injury. If it looks like there is going to be a problem, get anything sharp – from pencils to badges – off your person. Under extreme pressure a pen becomes a deadly weapon. Get rid of dentures and glasses too.

Check out the safety card. You may think that this makes you look like an inexperienced tourist, but the fact is that the information is there to increase your chances of survival. Planes do differ from model to model – don't take a risk by assuming that you know it all. A final precaution is to make sure you can find your flotation aid. In fact this is much less likely to be needed than a smoke hood (see the box below) – there are very few survivable crashes on water – but in the very unlikely event you do need to use it you want to be able to find it and get it on quickly.

Planning for survival

When you get the warning that something is going to happen, get a plan together in your mind. Your survival may depend on it. The majority of survivors of air crashes have been prepared with a plan in this way, though, as Jerry Schemmel's account (below) shows, the reality can never be fully anticipated. If you haven't got a smoke hood, get a handkerchief or a similar piece of cloth as wet as you can to provide some protection.

Get something over your head. Objects will be flying around on impact – your head is all too easy to damage. Use something like a pillow for protection. Then adopt a brace position. If there's a seat in front it's probably best to use the standard airline recommendation of crossed wrists, palms forward, cushioning your head against the seat. Slide your legs forward until they contact the seat or baggage, so they aren't flung around. Alternatively, cross your arms over your calves and grab your ankles.

Quick Tip: Smoke Hoods

One of the worst difficulties after an aircraft crash is smoke. Fires and smoke often kill more people than the crash itself. Until airlines decide that smoke hoods are just as valuable as life jackets, if you want one you will have to carry your own.

If you do decide to invest in a smoke hood (see Airsafe on page 326 for details on purchasing these), make sure that it is somewhere easily accessible during flight. And practise putting it on beforehand. These hoods can be quite tricky to get in place, and you could waste valuable seconds fighting with something unfamiliar.

The moment of truth

Following a crash landing, the first few seconds can be critical. In a state of shock, many surviving passengers will stay in their seats, waiting to be told what to do. You can't be sure that the cabin crew are able to give you instructions.

Even when they do, many passengers fail to respond. Fire and smoke will get worse. The threat of an explosion looms. A stampede of passengers could catch you at any moment. Don't wait: get out – out to an exit through the smoke-filled fuselage. Don't carry anything (you may have to consciously put something down that you have clung on to) – you will need your hands to help balance and pull yourself through any restrictions.

Keep your head as low as you can. The air will be more breathable lower down, and you will have a better chance of seeing the emergency lighting that should run along either side of the aisle to guide you. If you can't see the exits but these lights are on, the light colour should be different (red instead of white) when you are opposite an exit. In theory the air would be best of all if you crawled along the floor. In practice, though, there is too much danger of being trampled by other passengers. Walk but keep your head down. As you go, don't push any people in front of you. You won't get there any faster, and you may be hit by a desperate fellow evacuee.

Don't assume that every exit is operational, or that it is safe to leave the plane from an exit just because it is open. Depending on how the plane has landed, some exits could be obscured or jammed. Be prepared to backtrack, though your first check should be to see if the matching exit on the other side of the plane is accessible and operating. If the exit is clear, make sure there is some route to safety outside – a slide or the wing or a natural route. There could already be a fire outside, or a significant drop from the exit.

If you have reached one of the small emergency exits

and the door is still in place, try to throw it clear (watch out for people below). These doors are much heavier than they look – be prepared for considerable exertion. If your exit is on to the wing, slide down to the wing. There should be a non-slip walkway marked on the surface, but if in doubt proceed with your bottom low and either slide down the extended part of the wing (flaps) or jump carefully from the edge.

If your exit is a main door and it is not already open, follow the instructions on the door to get it open. Again, these doors are very heavy – it may take considerable effort to get the process started. If the emergency chute inflates, jump down into the slide feet first, arms folded across your

---

Quick Tip: **The Critical Few Seconds**

- *Take a deep breath.*

- *Act – don't sit and wait.*

- *Don't carry anything.*

- *Find a clear route.*

- *Head for the exit.*

- *Keep your head low.*

- *Don't push.*

- *Get out and get well away.*

chest. If it doesn't inflate you will have to use it to help you climb down.

Finally, get well away from the plane (and encourage those around you to do so). It is quite often the case that shocked passengers will manage to get out but then stand around in a daze. The plane probably still contains a considerable volume of highly flammable fuel – it could go up in a fireball, raining debris around it any time. As quickly as you can, put a considerable distance – up to half a kilometre if possible – between you and the wreck.

The real thing

One of the problems with facing a crash is that it is so unusual an experience. Most of us will never have spoken to anyone who has been through one, let alone have experienced one ourselves. It is difficult to imagine just what it is going to be like. About the best picture most of us have is Hollywood's glossy version – and anyone who has seen Hollywood's attempts to portray anything as straightforward as what London looks like or an English accent will have serious doubts about the reality content of a Hollywood plane crash.

Here is what it is really like, in the words of Jerry Schemmel, a sports administrator and broadcaster who in 1989 survived the crash of United Airlines Flight 232 from Denver to Chicago. An hour into the flight, the number-two engine in the DC-10 aircraft exploded causing a total failure of the plane's hydraulic systems. For the next forty-five minutes the crew managed to ease the plane along, controlling it through variation in the engine thrust. Unbelievably, they managed to get near to the airport in Sioux City, Iowa. With almost no control available on landing, the plane slammed into the runway, breaking up. Of the 296 on board, 112 died. Jerry Schemmel takes up the story:

[My] thoughts were interrupted by Captain Haynes, back on the PA system. He was reminding us that he would give us a command – 'Brace! Brace! Brace!' – in about two minutes, which would be about 30 seconds before landing. He didn't pull any punches. 'And folks, I'm not going to kid anybody, this is gonna be rough,' he concluded . . .

I knew we were getting close. And then the announcement came. Captain Haynes gave us our final instruction, the order to brace. The philosophizing, the preparation and the pondering – all that was over. Everything from here on out would be reaction to the unseen forces that would deliver all of us to our fate . . .

The wait dragged on: 'It's been more than 30 seconds,' I remember thinking to myself, and just as the thought formed in my head, we hit the ground.

How do I describe the impact? It felt, for lack of any comparable experience, exactly as you'd expect to feel if you'd dropped thousands of feet out of the sky and hit the ground. The sound matched the force of the jolt, seeming to come at once from both the inside and outside of my head. At that moment, there would have been no way to even subconsciously put words to the event, but the feeling in my gut was that this was no crash landing. In fact, this was no landing at all. It was simply an airplane slamming to earth.

For all the painful clutching of the seat back in front of me, my hands immediately lost their grip and my head, wedged against the same cushion, popped straight up like some character in an arcade game. The irresistible momentum moved me forward and upward from my seat until I had the sensation of floating in the air, held back only by my seat belt.

Gradually, the momentum slowed until I could feel myself easing back into my own seat cushions. Though my eyes were squeezed tightly shut, afraid to look at the havoc unfolding around me, I somehow became aware that the cabin lights went out. Screams cut through the thunderous sounds of the impact. I reached out to brace again against the seat back in front of me. My hands groped in the darkness but felt only a void; there was nothing there anymore. The seat in front of me was already gone. I tried in vain to clutch something, anything, to help fight the unbelievable force trying to wrench me out of my seat. But the crash had instantly rearranged the cabin in ways too horrible to imagine.

With no seat back to grab, I fumbled for my own arm rests and managed to pull myself back into my seat, as deep into the cushions as I could. For a split second I thought I was making headway, that I was winning this battle against the laws of physics; and then, in the next instant, I heard more screams and moans. I let my eyes open in the near darkness of the careening cabin and saw a human body fly past me, upside-down. A woman, still strapped in her seat, flew past me on the other side. A storm of debris seemed to whirl around me, as if I were sitting in the eye of a hurricane. When a ball of fire shot past on my right, from front to back of the cabin, I remember thinking it was just a matter of time before something hit me. I ducked my head and tried to cover my face. For all my mental preparation for this moment there was nothing left to do but react instinctively to the raw physical chaos. It was a helpless feeling, a sensation of total vulnerability.

Once again, time moved in slow, elastic increments. The plane, too, seemed to be slowing slightly, though in reality it was still screaming across the ground at a frightening clip. But there was a steadiness in the motion, and the thought occurred that the worst was over, that we would simply coast to a stop and – miracle of miracles – I might even walk away from this experience. That's when we flipped over.

A sharp pain rippled through my back as I felt myself, still strapped into my seat, roll forward with the pitch of the cabin. A tremendous burning sensation that started in my lower back and travelled quickly up my spine to the back of my neck made me wonder, momentarily, if I'd been electrocuted.

A moment later, I hung upside down in my seat, waiting for the momentum of the roll to right us. But it never did.

When the aircraft finally jolted to a halt, Schemmel tells of a terrible scene:

Slowly my eyes adjusted to what remained of our portion of the cabin, lighted mostly by flames. Where I had minutes earlier made note of an emergency exit stood twisted, burning steel. Where Georgia, the flight attendant, had been sitting there was only a wall of fire. 'She's dead,' I thought. 'Forget about her. Move on.'

For the first time since the impact the concept of death, the reality of human casualties, hit home – though I would later learn that Georgia had survived. The horrible toll struck me much more vividly as I turned and scanned the rest of the cabin. Even in the dim light and gathering smoke the scene was shocking.

Dozens of people remained strapped in their seats, still upside-down. Some were struggling to break free. Others were hanging limp and lifeless. From one dangling passenger, blood trickled to the floor. From another still body, it poured in a steady stream. And from yet another lifeless form, an arm hung by a thread while flames consumed the rest. Bodies were strewn across the ceiling, now the floor of the airplane. Some moved. Many did not. Seats had collapsed, row by row, and been flattened. Yet, incredibly, shadowy figures also moved about, on their feet, in the smoky light. That scene, that first conscious glimpse of what United 232 had wrought, would never go away. It would appear over and over again in nightmares.

To get the full picture of this remarkable story, see Schemmel's moving book *Chosen to Live* (Victory Publishing Company, Littleton Co., USA). He portrays a frightening scene, with the presence of fire and smoke as much (if not more) of a threat than the impact itself. Many people lost their lives in this terrible accident. Yet Schemmel did survive, as did 184 others. There may not be much consolation in this terrifying description, but if there is some it is that so many people could survive such a violent landing. Hope is always there.

✈ *Summary:* Crash Landing – Surviving the Unthinkable

- Every month there are hundreds of incidents that seem life-threatening to the passengers but prove harmless.

- The survival rate for air crashes is above 50 per cent.

- Making basic preparation for survival – envisaging your route to the exit and wearing sensible clothes – can make a lot of difference.

- When you get the warning that something is going to happen, establish a survival plan in your mind.

- Take a deep breath and orient yourself.

- Get out as quickly as you can without running.

- Keep your head low to avoid smoke.

- Get well away from the plane.

17 Making the Most of It

It's easy to turn flying into a chore, especially when we are bombarded with health scares and stories of bad customer service. I hope that this book has enabled you to put the risks into proportion – not to ignore what can go wrong, but to be prepared for the worse without spoiling what can often be an enjoyable experience.

The appendices

The remainder of the book is a series of appendices, providing a source of reference to expand the information available to the flier. Most of the content has been chosen to remain reasonably constant, but the airline world is fast-changing, so perhaps the most useful of the sections is Appendix 5 (page 323), which contains web links to provide the most up-to-date information.

You want more?

If you feel that anything is missing from *The Complete Flier's Handbook*, or would like to go further into any point mentioned in the book, please drop me an e-mail at fliers@cul.co.uk

Appendix 1 The jabs

What are they?

The following immunizations are commonly recommended to travellers. Try to have your inoculations done six to eight weeks in advance. Most boosters are effective immediately, but an initial inoculation may need this long to take effect. Others typically take two weeks for the initial impact.

A few of the immunizations themselves have negative side effects. To overcome the side-effects some travellers have used homoeopathic remedies. Others use homoeopathy as an alternative to immunization. The alternative approaches may work, but those who take such remedies must be aware that they are opening themselves up to potentially life-threatening diseases without proven protection. See page 328 for web sites of homoeopathic pharmacies. Always consult a medical doctor before resorting to alternatives to immunization.

Cholera

Cholera is an uncommon disease in travellers. The injected vaccine was of poor efficacy and is no longer available in the UK. Immunization against cholera is not appropriate for most travellers, although, where it is known that border officials may demand a cholera certificate, stating your country of origin is cholera-free, it is wiser to be in possession of such a certificate prior to departure.

Hepatitis A

Short-term protection against this water-borne viral disease is offered by a single injection of immunoglobulin. A vaccine is now available which provides protection for ten years and is suitable for the frequent traveller. Immunization is usually advised for those going to areas where the standards of food and water hygiene are lower than in the UK. A booster is required at six months to ensure the full ten years' protection.

Polio

This vaccine is given orally, and is a simple and safe protection against poliomyelitis, which is still prevalent in tropical and developing countries. It used to be given on a sugar lump, but this is now usually omitted so as to be more tooth-friendly. A booster is needed every ten years.

Tetanus

Everyone, travellers and others, should be up to date for tetanus immunization, as the disease is spread throughout the world and is potentially a hazard to life. Initial protection is by a series of three injections; a booster dose is given as a single injection and lasts for ten years.

Typhoid

Typhoid is a disease contracted from contaminated food and water, and leads to high fever and septicaemia. There are now three vaccines for protection against typhoid: the older monovalent vaccine (no longer available in the UK), a new injected single-dose vaccine, and a live oral vaccine. Immunization is usually advised for those going to areas where the standards of food and water hygiene are lower than in the UK.

Yellow fever

A single injection provides protection against yellow fever for ten years. An International Certificate of Vaccination against Yellow Fever is valid from ten days after the injection or immediately upon revaccination, and is a mandatory requirement for entry into certain countries (see below).

*

appendix 1

The following vaccinations are sometimes recommended for those at special risk or who are liable to be in an infected area for a long period of time.

Diphtheria

Most travellers from the UK will have been immunized against diphtheria in childhood. A booster of low-dose vaccine would be advised every ten years for those intending to make long-stay trips to developing countries. Travellers to the former Soviet Union should be in date for diphtheria, as there is an epidemic of this disease at the time of writing.

Travellers also requiring a booster for tetanus should be given the new combined diphtheria/tetanus vaccine.

Hepatitis B

Hepatitis B is a viral disease of the liver that is endemic in many tropical countries. It is transmitted by sexual activity and through contaminated needles and syringes. Travellers at particular risk should consider being in date for this immunization. The course comprises two injections separated by one month, and a further injection at six months. An accelerated schedule is available for those who do not have time to complete the recommended course.

Japanese encephalitis

Japanese encephalitis is a serious viral disease transmitted by mosquitoes in certain rural parts of India, Asia and South-East Asia. A vaccine is available, which should be reserved for those going to risk areas for periods of a month or more.

Meningococcal meningitis

A single-dose vaccine is available which protects against the A and C strains of meningococcal meningitis and is advised for travellers to areas where there are outbreaks of these strains of the disease. Long-stay travellers to areas where the disease is endemic (e.g. the 'meningitis belt' in northern sub-Saharan Africa in the dry season) should also be offered the vaccine. A booster is required every three to five years.

Rabies

Immunization against rabies should be considered by travellers going to areas where rabies is endemic or who are staying for considerable periods of time. The immunization should not be considered to provide complete protection, and medical advice must be sought if bitten by a potentially rabid animal. Remember that this could be a seemingly friendly species – in the USA, for example, rabies is common among racoons.

Tick-borne encephalitis (European)

Tick-borne encephalitis is a viral disease transmitted by ticks. It is prevalent in certain European countries, where the ticks are found in the long grass at the edge of forests. The vaccine is recommended for those who will be staying in such areas for prolonged periods of time.

Tuberculosis (TB)

The majority of travellers from the UK will have had a BCG vaccination in childhood and do not need to be boosted. Unimmunized adults and children spending prolonged periods in areas where TB is endemic should consider immunization. The vaccine is given as a single injection. For those over three months of age it is important that a test is performed before giving the vaccine. This test (usually a Heaf test) checks for existing immunity to TB.

What immunization do I need?

Please note, the table below offers only general guidelines; advice should be taken for an individual itinerary. This Crown Copyright material originally appeared on the UK Department of Health web site at www.doh.gov.uk/travel-advice, and is reproduced with the permission of the Controller of Her Majesty's Stationery Office.

The following symbols are used in the table:

➤ Immunization is an essential requirement for entry to the country concerned and you will require a certificate.

➤1 Immunization is essential except for infants under one year (but note the advice above).

➤2 Immunization is essential (except for infants under one year) unless arriving from non-infected areas and staying for less than two weeks. The UK is a non-infected area, but seek medical advice if travelling via Equatorial Africa or South America.

➤3 Immunization is essential if the traveller arrives from an infected country or area (this will not apply if your journey is direct from the UK). The age limit below which this does not apply varies.

➤4 Immunization is essential if arriving within six days of having visited an infected country.

✔ Immunization or tablets are recommended for protection against disease, but note that, for yellow fever, pregnant women and infants under nine months should not normally be immunized and therefore should avoid exposure to infection.

[✔] Depends on area visited.

D Check that immunized against diphtheria.

M Meningitis vaccination advised, depending on the area visited and the time of year.

No special immunizations are required for those European countries not listed.

Country	Hep. A, polio, typhoid*	Malaria	Yellow fever	Other
Afghanistan	✔	✔	➢3	
Albania	✔		➢3	
Algeria	✔		➢3	
Andorra				
Angola	✔	✔	➢3	
Anguilla	✔			
Antigua and Barbuda	✔		➢3	
Argentina	✔	[✔]		
Armenia	✔			
Aruba	✔			
Ascension Islands				
Australia			➢4	
Azerbaijan	✔	[✔]		
Bahamas	✔		➢3	

Country	Hep. A, polio, typhoid*	Malaria	Yellow fever	Other
Bahrain	✔			
Bali	✔		≻3	
Bangladesh	✔	✔	≻4	
Barbados	✔		≻3	
Belarus	✔			
Belize	✔	✔	≻3	
Benin	✔	✔	≻1	M
Bermuda	✔			
Bhutan		[✔]	≻3	M
Bolivia	✔	✔	≻3 ✔	
Borneo	✔	[✔]	≻3	
Bosnia-Hercegovina	✔			
Botswana	✔	[✔]		
Brazil	✔	✔	≻3 ✔	
Brunei	✔		≻4	
Bulgaria	✔			
Burkina Faso	✔	✔	≻1	M
Burma – see Myanmar				

Country	Hep. A, polio, typhoid*	Malaria	Yellow fever	Other
Burundi	✔	✔	⪴3 ✔	M
Cambodia	✔	✔	⪴3	
Cameroon	✔	✔	⪴1	M
Canada				
Cape Verde	✔	Limited risk in São Tiàgo Island	⪴3 ✔	
Cayman Islands	✔			
Central African Republic	✔	✔	⪴1	M
Chad	✔	✔	⪴1	M
Chile	✔			
China	✔	[✔]	⪴3	M
Colombia	✔	✔	✔	
Comoros	✔	✔		
Cook Islands	✔			
Costa Rica	✔	[✔]		
Croatia	✔			
Cuba	✔			
Cyprus				

Country	Hep. A, polio, typhoid*	Malaria	Yellow fever	Other
Czech and Slovak Republics	✔			
Democratic Republic of Congo (Zaire)	✔	✔	≻1	
Djibouti	✔	✔	≻3 ✔	M
Dominica	✔		≻3	
Dominican Republic	✔	✔		
Ecuador	✔	✔	≻3 ✔	
Egypt	✔	[✔]	≻3	
El Salvador	✔	✔	≻3	
Equatorial Guinea	✔	✔	≻3 ✔	
Eritrea	✔	✔	≻3	M
Estonia	✔	✔	≻3 ✔	M
Ethiopia	✔		≻3	
Falkland Islands				
Fiji	✔		≻3	
French Guiana	✔	✔	≻1	
French Polynesia (Tahiti)	✔		≻3	

Country	Hep. A, polio, typhoid*	Malaria	Yellow fever	Other
Gabon	✔	✔	≻1	
The Gambia	✔	✔	≻3 ✔	M
Georgia	✔			
Ghana	✔	✔	≻1	M
Greece			≻3	
Greenland				
Grenada	✔		≻3	
Guadeloupe	✔		≻3	
Guam	✔			
Guatemala	✔	✔	≻3	
Guinea	✔	✔	≻3 ✔	M
Guinea-Bissau	✔	✔	≻3 ✔	M
Guyana	✔	✔	≻3 ✔	
Haiti	✔	✔	≻3	
Honduras	✔	✔	≻3	
Hong Kong	✔			
Hungary				
India	✔	✔	≻4	M

Country	Hep. A, polio, typhoid*	Malaria	Yellow fever	Other
Indonesia	✔	[✔]	➢3	
Iran	✔	✔	➢3	
Iraq	✔	[✔]	➢3	
Israel	✔			
Ivory Coast	✔	✔	➢1	M
Jamaica	✔		➢3	
Japan	✔	✔		
Jordan	✔		➢3	
Kazakhstan	✔		➢3	
Kenya	✔	✔	➢3 ✔	M
Kiribati	✔		➢3	
Kirzigstan	✔			
Korea (North and South)	✔			
Kuwait	✔			
Laos	✔	✔	➢3	
Latvia				
Lebanon	✔		➢3	
Lesotho	✔		➢3	

Country	Hep. A, polio, typhoid*	Malaria	Yellow fever	Other
Liberia	✔	✔	≻1	M
Libya	✔		≻3	
Lithuania				
Macau	✔			
Macedonia	✔			
Madagascar	✔	✔	≻3	
Madeira			≻3	
Malawi	✔	✔	≻3	M
Malaysia	✔	[✔]	≻3	
Maldives	✔		≻3	
Mali	✔	✔	≻1	M
Malta			≻3	
Marshall Islands	✔			
Martinique	✔		≻3	
Mauritania	✔	✔	≻2	
Mauritius	✔	[✔]	≻3	
Mayotte	✔	✔		
Mexico	✔	[✔]	≻3	

Country	Hep. A, polio, typhoid*	Malaria	Yellow fever	Other
Federated States of Micronesia	✔			
Moldova	✔			
Monaco				
Mongolia	✔			
Montserrat	✔			
Morocco	✔			
Mozambique	✔	✔	≥3	M
Myanmar (Burma)	✔	✔	≥3	
Namibia	✔	[✔]	≥3	
Nauru	✔		≥3	
Nepal	✔	✔	≥3	M
Netherlands Antilles	✔		≥3	
New Caledonia	✔		≥3	
New Zealand				
Nicaragua	✔	✔	≥3	
Niger	✔	✔	≥1	M
Nigeria	✔	✔	≥3 ✔	M
Niue	✔		≥3	

Country	Hep. A, polio, typhoid*	Malaria	Yellow fever	Other
Northern Mariana Islands	✔			
Oman	✔	✔	➢3	
Pakistan	✔	✔		M
Palau	✔	✔		
Panama	✔	✔	Recommended for Province of Darién	
Papua New Guinea	✔	✔	➢3	
Paraguay	✔	✔	➢3 Certificate required if leaving Paraguay for endemic areas	
Peru	✔	✔	➢3 ✔	
Philippines	✔	[✔]	➢3	
Pitcairn Island	✔		➢3	
Poland				
Puerto Rico	✔			
Qatar	✔			
Réunion	✔		➢3	
Romania	✔			

Country	Hep. A, polio, typhoid*	Malaria	Yellow fever	Other
Russia				D
Rwanda	✔		≻1	M
St Helena	✔		≻3	
St Kitts and Nevis	✔		≻3	
St Lucia	✔		≻3	
St Vincent and Grenadines	✔		≻3	
Samoa	✔		≻3	
São Tomé and Príncipe	✔		≻1	
Saudi Arabia	✔		≻3	M
Senegal	✔		≻3 ✔	M
Seychelles	✔		≻4	
Sierra Leone	✔		≻3 ✔	M
Singapore	✔		≻4	
Slovenia	✔			
Solomon Islands	✔		≻3	
Somalia	✔		≻3 ✔	M
South Africa	✔		≻3	
Sri Lanka	✔		≻3	

Country	Hep. A, polio, typhoid*	Malaria	Yellow fever	Other
Sudan	✔		⋗3 ✔	M
Surinam	✔		⋗3 ✔	
Swaziland	✔		⋗3	
Switzerland				
Syria	✔		⋗3	
Taiwan	✔		⋗3	
Tajikistan	✔			D
Tanzania	✔		⋗3 ✔	M
Thailand	✔		⋗3	
Togo	✔		⋗1	M
Tokelau	✔			
Tonga	✔		⋗3	
Trinidad and Tobago	✔		⋗3	
Tristan de Cunha	✔			
Tunisia	✔		⋗3	
Turkey	✔			
Turkmenistan	✔			
Turks and Caicos Islands				

Country	Hep. A, polio, typhoid*	Malaria	Yellow fever	Other
Tuvalu	✔			
Uganda	✔	✔	≻3 ✔	M
Ukraine				D
United Arab Emirates	✔	[✔]		
Uruguay	✔			
USA				
Uzbekistan	✔			
Vanuatu	✔	✔		
Venezuela	✔	✔	✔	
Vietnam	✔	[✔]	≻3	
Virgin Islands	✔			
Wallis and Futana Islands	✔			
West Indies	✔		≻3	
Yemen	✔	✔	≻3	
Yugoslavia	✔			
Zambia	✔	✔	✔	
Zimbabwe	✔	[✔]	≻3	

* Immunization against typhoid may be less important for short stays in first-class conditions

Appendix 2 Emergency Medical Kits

An emergency medical kit to assist the medical team in countries with poor medical facilities provides peace of mind. Kits can be bought from pharmacists or travel clinics, or direct from the suppliers. Ensure that the kit is sealed and has appropriate documentation to keep customs officials happy. Kits are also obtainable from travel clinics – contact British Airways travel clinics (phone 01276 685040, web site http://www.britishairways.com/travelclinics), or the Medical Advisory Service for Travellers Abroad run by the London School of Hygiene and Tropical Medicine (www.masta.org).

✔ *Check List: Medical Kits*
  There are some low-value kits on the market that simply won't deliver the necessary goods. To be worthwhile, a kit should contain a minimum of:

  ❏ Two syringes (5 ml)
  ❏ Five needles (ideally two sizes)
  ❏ Dental needle

- Intravenous cannula
- Skin suture with needle
- Packet of skin closure strips
- Five alcohol swabs for skin cleansing
- Non-stick dressings (5-cm square and 10-cm square)
- Roll of surgical tape

For more remote locations you might also like to carry:

- Intravenous blood-giving set
- Blood-substitute solution

Appendix 3 Airline Safety Records

The columns in the tables below refer to:

- *Flights* – number of flights since 1970 in millions.

- *Events* – number of flights involving fatalities among the passengers.

- *Last* – last time a flight involved a fatal event.

- *FLE* – 'Full Loss Equivalent'. The fraction of passengers killed for each event is added together. If there was one crash with half the passengers killed and another with 10 out of 100, the FLE would be 0.5+0.1, i.e. 0.6. This is a factor which then reflects the seriousness of the event.

- *Score* – the FLE divided by the number of flights in millions. This gives a feel for the safety level of the airline. The larger the number, the more doubtful the safety. However, bear in mind that 0 gives no indication of how few flights have been undertaken.

Highest-scoring airlines

Small variations of score are of no significance in reflecting airline safety, but these particularly high-scoring companies have to be regarded with some suspicion. Airlines with incomplete information have been included at the top – this does not mean that they are necessarily high-scoring, though some, like the airlines of the former Soviet Union, almost certainly are.

Airline	Flights	Events	Last	FLE	Score
Airlines of the former Soviet Union	?	18	2001	13.26	?
Ansett of New Zealand	?	1	1995	0.22	?
Austral Lineas Aereas	?	4	1997	4	?
Gulf Air	?	2	2000	1.95	?
Other People's Republic of China Airlines	?	14	1999	7.28	?
Thai Airways Company	?	3	1987	2.82	?
Cubana	0.33	8	1999(2)	6.11	18.53
Air Zimbabwe	0.16	2	1979	1.85	11.54
AeroPeru	0.12	2	1996	1.17	9.74
Royal Jordanian	0.34	3	1979	2.72	7.99
EgyptAir/Air Sinai	0.75	6	1999	5.5	7.33

Airline	Flights	Events	Last	FLE	Score
China Airlines (Taiwan)	0.90	9	1999	5.44	6.04
THY	1.10	8	1994	6.51	5.92
AirTran (ValuJet)	0.17	1	1996	1	5.88
TAM	0.60	5	1997	3.4	5.67
Air India	0.44	3	1985	2.15	4.89

Fatal-event rates by airline since 1970

Airline	Flights	Events	Last	FLE	Score
Aer Lingus/Aer Lingus Commuter	1.20	0	–	0	0
Aeroflot and other airlines of the former Soviet Union	?	18	2001	13.26	?
Aerolineas Argentinas	1.67	2	1992	1.01	0.6
Aeromexico	2.16	4	1986	3.8	1.76
AeroPeru	0.12	2	1996	1.17	9.74
Air Afrique	0.30	1	1987	0.01	0.02
Air Canada	4.75	3	1983	1.58	0.33
Air China	?	0	–	0	0
Air France/Air France Europe	5.90	7	2000	3.23	0.55
Air India	0.44	3	1985	2.15	4.89

Airline	Flights	Events	Last	FLE	Score
Air Jamaica	0.29	0	–	0	0
Air New Zealand	1.35	1	1979	1	0.74
Air Zimbabwe	0.16	2	1979	1.85	11.54
AirTran (ValuJet)	0.17	1	1996	1	5.88
Alaska Airlines/Horizon Air	4.05	3	2000	2.02	0.5
Alitalia	3.90	3	1990	2.83	0.73
All Nippon Airways	4.64	1	1971	1	0.22
Allegro Airlines	?	0	–	0	0
Aloha Airlines/Aloha Islandair	1.34	1	1989	1	0.75
America West Airlines	2.30	0	–	0	0
American Airlines/American Eagle	17.0	9	1999	6.23	0.37
American Trans Air	0.33	0	–	0	0
Ansett Australia	?	0	–	0	0
Ansett of New Zealand	?	1	1995	0.22	?
Asiana Airlines	0.54	1	1993	0.62	1.14
Austral Lineas Aereas	?	4	1997	4	?
Austrian Airlines	0.75	0	–	0	0
Avianca	1.27	4	1990	3.82	3.01
Braathens	1.35	1	1972	0.88	0.65

Airline	Flights	Events	Last	FLE	Score
British Airways	6.35	2	1985	1.4	0.22
British Midland Airways	1.03	1	1989	0.4	0.39
BWIA West Indies Airways	0.45	0	–	0	0
Canadian Airlines	?	0	–	0	0
Cathay Pacific	0.69	1	1972	1	1.45
China Airlines (Taiwan)	0.90	9	1999	5.44	6.04
Continental Airlines/Continental Express	8.0	5	1997	1.47	0.18
Cubana	0.33	8	1999(2)	6.11	18.53
Delta Airlines/Delta Connection	20.0	6	1997	3.24	0.16
EgyptAir/Air Sinai	0.75	6	1999	5.5	7.33
El Al	0.34	0	–	0	0
Emirates	?	0	–	0	0
Ethiopian Airlines	0.50	2	1996	1.03	2.06
EVA Air	?	0	–	0	0
Finnair	1.70	0	–	0	0
Garuda Indonesia Airlines	1.96	8	1997	4.78	2.44
Gulf Air	?	2	2000	1.95	?
Hawaiian Airlines	0.33	0	–	0	0
Iberia	4.50	4	1985	3.6	0.8

Airline	Flights	Events	Last	FLE	Score
Icelandair	0.39	0	–	0	0
Indian Airlines	2.50	12	1999	8.82	3.53
Iran Air	0.80	2	1988	2	2.5
Japan Air Lines	2.44	5	1985	3.31	1.36
Japan Air System	?	0	–	0	0
JetBlue Airlines	?	0	–	0	0
Kenya Airways	0.33	1	2000	0.94	2.85
KLM/KLM Cityhopper	2.40	3	1994	1.94	0.81
Korean Air	1.30	7	1997	3.35	2.58
Kuwait Airways	0.35	0	–	0	0
LAN Chile	0.50	2	1991	0.34	0.68
Lufthansa/Condor	7.30	3	1993	1.41	0.19
Malaysia Airlines	1.80	2	1995	1.65	0.92
Mexicana	1.90	1	1986	1	0.53
Midway Airlines	0.08	0	–	0	0
Midwest Express	0.26	1	1985	1	3.85
Nigeria Airways	0.60	3	1995	1.84	3.07
Northwest Airlines/Northwest Airline	9.2	4	1993	2.61	0.28
Olympic Airways/Olympic Aviation	1.80	3	1989	2.73	1.52

Airline	Flights	Events	Last	FLE	Score
Other People's Republic of China Airlines	?	14	1999	7.28	?
Pakistan International Airlines	1.40	7	1992	5.37	3.84
Philippine Air Lines	1.71	8	1994	4.23	2.47
Qantas	1.02	0	–	0	0
Royal Air Maroc	0.65	1	1994	1	1.54
Royal Jordanian	0.34	3	1979	2.72	7.99
Sabena	1.60	0	–	0	0
SAS	5.40	0	–	0	0
Saudi Arabian Airlines	2.15	3	1996	2.01	0.93
Singapore Airlines/SilkAir	1.00	2	2000	1.5	1.5
South African Airways	1.60	1	1987	1	0.63
Southwest Airlines	9.50	0	–	0	0
Swissair/Crossair	3.20	4	2000	3.1	0.97
TACA	0.25	0	–	0	0
TAESA	0.35	1	1999	1	2.86
TAM	0.60	5	1997	3.4	5.67
TAP Air Portugal	0.85	1	1977	0.8	0.94
Thai Airways Company	?	3	1987	2.82	?
Thai Airways International	1.05	2	1998	1.68	1.6

Airline	Flights	Events	Last	FLE	Score
THY	1.10	8	1994	6.51	5.92
Tower Air	0.03	0	–	0	0
Transbrasil	0.85	2	1980	1.77	2.09
Tunis Air	0.30	0	–	0	0
TWA/Trans World Express	8.10	6	1996	3.05	0.38
United Airlines/United Express	18.0	9	1997	4.69	0.26
US Airways/USAir Express	14.3	8	1994	3.97	0.28
VASP	1.85	6	1986	3.34	1.81
Varig	2.45	3	1989	2.22	0.9
Virgin Atlantic	0.05	0	–	0	0

Data for all statistics were obtained from the International Civil Aviation Organization, the Federal Aviation Administration, the US National Transportation Safety Board and the US Department of Transportation. This table is reproduced by kind permission of Todd Curtis and Airsafe (www.airsafe.com).

While every effort has been made to check these figures, we cannot guarantee accuracy, or endorse commercial decisions based on them. Safety statistics are to early 2001.

Appendix 4 The Safest Planes to Fly

The columns in the tables below refer to:

- *Flights* – number of flights since 1970 in millions.

- *Events* – number of flights involving fatalities among the passengers.

- *FLE* – 'Full Loss Equivalent'. The fraction of passengers killed for each event is added together. If there was one crash with half the passengers killed and another with 10 out of 100, the FLE would be 0.5+0.1, i.e. 0.6. This is a factor which then reflects the seriousness of the event.

- *Rate* – the number of events divided by the number of flights in millions. This gives a feel for the safety of the aircraft in terms of chances of something going wrong. The larger the number, the more doubtful the safety – but bear in mind that 0 gives no indication of how few flights were flown.

- *Score* – the FLE divided by the number of flights in millions. This gives a feel for the overall safety level of the aircraft, taking into account the seriousness of the events. The larger the number, the more doubtful the safety. However, bear in mind that 0 gives no indication of how few flights have been undertaken.

Aircraft with highest rates

The following aircraft seem most likely to have a fatal event. Note that Concorde is a special case, as it has flown so few flights compared with a typical airliner. Some aircraft where the number of flights is unknown have been included – this doesn't mean that these are more dangerous, but there are particular doubts about aircraft of the former Soviet Union, which aren't listed here.

Model	Flights	Events	FLE	Rate	Score
British Aerospace Jetstream	?	6	5.22	?	?
Dornier 228	?	7	6.88	?	?
Dornier 328	?	1	0.11	?	?
Concorde	0.08	1	1	12.5	12.5
Boeing MD11	0.8	3	1.02	3.75	1.27
Embraer Bandeirante	7.5	28	23	3.73	3.07
Fokker F28	8.1	20	14.45	2.47	1.78

Aircraft with highest scores

The following aircraft seem to have been the most dangerous. Note that Concorde is a special case, as it has flown
so few flights compared with a typical airliner. Some aircraft
where the number of flights is unknown have been included
– this doesn't mean that these are more dangerous, but
there are particular doubts about aircraft of the former
Soviet Union, which aren't listed here.

Model	Flights	Events	FLE	Rate	Score
British Aerospace Jetstream	?	6	5.22	?	?
Dornier 228	?	7	6.88	?	?
Dornier 328	?	1	0.11	?	?
Concorde	0.08	1	1	12.5	12.5
Embraer Bandeirante	7.8	28	23	3.73	3.07
Fokker F28	8.1	20	14.45	2.47	1.78
Airbus A310	2.9	5	4.62	1.72	1.59
Boeing MD11	0.8	3	1.02	3.75	1.27

Fatal events since 1959

Model	Flights	Events	FLE	Rate	Score
Airbus A300	7.7	8	4.99	1.04	0.65
Airbus A310	2.9	5	4.62	1.72	1.59
Airbus A320	7.3	5	2.61	0.68	0.38
ATR	3.2	3	3	0.94	0.94
Boeing 727	72.2	46	35.34	0.64	0.49
Boeing 737-100/200	50.4	37	26.29	0.73	0.52
Boeing 737-300/400/500	30.8	10	8.76	0.32	0.28
Boeing 737 (all models)	81.2	47	35.05	0.58	0.43
Boeing 747	13.1	25	12.73	1.91	0.97
Boeing 757	8.7	5	3.4	0.57	0.39
Boeing 767	7.3	3	2.73	0.41	0.37
Boeing 777	0.7	0	0	0	0
Boeing DC9	58.1	42	34.41	0.72	0.59
Boeing DC10	7.8	15	5.91	1.92	0.76
Boeing MD11	0.8	3	1.02	3.75	1.27
Boeing MD80/MD90	23.3	8	4.19	0.34	0.18
British Aerospace BAe 146	5.4	4	2.81	0.74	0.52

appendix 4

Airline	Flights	Events	FLE	Rate	Score
British Aerospace Jetstream	?	6	5.22	?	?
Concorde	0.08	1	1	12.5	12.5
Dornier 228	?	7	6.88	?	?
Dornier 328	?	1	0.11	?	?
Embraer Bandeirante	7.5	28	23	3.73	3.07
Embraer Brasilia	7.4	5	4.27	0.68	0.58
Fokker F28	8.1	20	14.45	2.47	1.78
Fokker F70/F100	3.8	3	1.86	0.79	0.49
Lockheed L1011	5.2	5	2.54	0.96	0.49
Saab 340	9.7	3	2.1	0.31	0.22

Flight numbers were computed using data from Boeing's *Statistical Summary of Commercial Jet Airplane Accidents: 1959–1999*. This table is reproduced by kind permission of Todd Curtis and Airsafe (www.airsafe.com).

While every effort has been made to check these figures, we cannot guarantee accuracy, or endorse commercial decisions made based on them. Safety statistics are to early 2001.

Appendix 5 Fliers Online

Airlines

Most airline sites will allow you to check timetables and prices and book seats online. With the major airlines you can also see seat maps of the planes to find out just where 23C is located, and even check out the movies that will be showing on the flight.

The following isn't a definitive list of airline web sites, but covers many of the major airlines. If the carrier you want isn't listed, try www.*x*.com, where *x* is the airline's name, or enter the airline's name into a search engine like www.altavista.com.

- Aer Lingus – www.aerlingus.ie

- Air Canada – www.aircanada.ca

- Air France – www.airfrance.co.uk

- Air India – www.airindia.com

- Air New Zealand – www.airnz.com

- Alaska Air – www.alaskaair.com

- Alitalia – www.alitalia.it/eng

- American Airlines – www.aa.com

- British Airways – www.british-airways.com

- British Midland – www.flybmi.com

- Continental Airlines – www.flycontinental.com

- Delta Airlines – www.delta-air.com

- Easyjet – www.easyjet.com

- Japan Airlines – www.jal.co.jp

- Lufthansa – www.lufthansa.de

- Pakistan International – www.piac.com

- Qantas – www.qantas.com

- Northwest Airlines – www.nwa.com

- Sabena – www.sabena.com

- SAS – www.sas.se

- Singapore Airlines – www.sinaporeair.com

- Southwest Airlines – www.southwest.com

- Swissair – www.swissair.com

- TWA – www.twa.com

- United Airlines – www.ual.com

- US Air – www.usair.com

- Virgin Atlantic Airways – www.virginatlantic.com

Alliances

Many airlines are getting together to share frequent-flier miles and other benefits. These web sites belong to the big four:

- OneWorld – www.oneworld.com

- Skyteam – www.skyteam.com

- Star – www.star-alliance.com

- Northwest Airlines/KLM – www.nwa.com/alliance

Timetabling and ticketing web sites

If you don't want to deal direct with an airline, there are a range of sites providing cross-carrier information and ticketing, often at a substantial discount. Some, like Expedia, provide all-round travel sites. Others, such as Dial A Flight, are very much focused on cheap tickets. The choice is yours.

- Deckchair – www.deckchair.com

- Dial A Flight – www.dialaflight.com

- Excite Travel – travel.excite.com

- Expedia – www.expedia.com

- Farebase – www.farebase.net

- Netflights – www.netflights.com

- OAG (the oldest cross-airline source) – www.oag.com

- Yahoo Travel – www.travel.yahoo.com

General flying sites

Note that I can't guarantee the quality of information at any of the following sites, and it is possible that they may contain information that is contradictory to the information in this book – that's the joy of the Internet.

- Airsafe – a site dedicated to airline safety, with lots of useful information and safety-based products – www.airsafe.com

- Air Transport Users Council – the UK passengers' watchdog – www.auc.org.uk

- Aviation Now – the web site of the industry magazine *Aviation Week* – www.aviationnow.com

- Baby B'Air – manufacturers of in-flight harnesses for babies and toddlers – www.babybair.com

- Fliertalk – bulletin boards for discussing every aspect of flying – ideal if there's a specific question you'd like to ask – www.fliertalk.com

- Flight Safety Foundation – an organization specializing in the academic end of the study of flight safety – www.flightsafety.org

- Flight Source – general information about air travel and flight and hotel information – www.flightsource.net

- Foreign and Commonwealth Office (UK) – lots of guidance and quick identification of the danger spots – www.fco.gov.uk/travel/

- Inside Flier – an online magazine for users of frequent-flier programmes – www.insideflier.com

- Department for Environment, Food and Rural Affairs (UK) – information on pet passports – www.defra.gov.uk/animalh/quarantine

- Passport Agency (UK) – www.ukpa.gov.uk

- Points.com – everything you ever wanted to know about frequent-flier schemes, and a unique points-exchange programme too – www.points.com

- State Department (US) – like the UK Foreign Office, plenty of guidance on danger spots, but with a slightly different slant – www.travel.state.gov/

- Worldwise – an excellent guide to what's what in different destinations – www.brookes.ac.uk/worldwise/home.html

Aviation health sites

As with the general sites, I cannot provide any guarantees about the quality of information provided at the following sites.

- Ainsworths Homeopathic Pharmacy – homoeopathic medication for travellers – www.ainsworths.com

- Aviation Health Institute (UK) – general information, and sells air-filter masks – www.aviation-health.org

- British Airways Travel Clinics – www.britishairways.com/ travelqa/fyi/health/health.shtml

- Flyana – the very personal site of ex-stewardess Diana Fairechild – www.flyana.com

- Health and Safety Executive (UK) – radiation-level test facilities – www.hse.gov.uk

- Helios Homoeopathic Pharmacy – www.helios.co.uk

- International Society of Travel Medicine – a very useful list of travel clinics around the world – www.istm.org/

- MASTA – Medical Advisory Service for Travellers Abroad – www.masta.org

Other sites of interest

- NOAA – US National Oceanic and Atmospheric Agency (solar-flare forecasts) – www.sec.noaa.gov

- NRPB – UK National Radiological Protection Board, providing information and support on radiation exposure and protection – www.nrpb.org

- Space Weather Bureau – lots of information on the sun's impact on the earth, including up-to-date forecasts of solar flares – www.spaceweather.com

Appendix 6 Don't Take It

Most airline tickets are covered in lists of items not to take on board. This is not bureaucracy run wild – airlines are just as enthusiastic as you are that the plane you are on is not hijacked and that it doesn't crash. Next time you feel like complaining that you can't take your favourite hunting knife with you, remember this. The following gives a good idea of the items to avoid, but can't be guaranteed to be complete – and of course the list changes from time to time.

Corrosives

Anything that is going to make a hole in the airframe or weaken the structure of the aircraft is bad news. Specifically, acids, alkaline substances, batteries with acid (like car batteries), drain cleaners and mercury (even in a thermometer) should not be carried.

Explosives

It should be obvious that you don't want an explosive on board a plane. To say that the airline and airport authorities are twitchy on the subject would be an understatement. Specifically, ammunition, blasting caps and charges, fireworks, flares, gunpowder, matches and sparklers should be avoided.

Flammable substances

Although a fire on board an aircraft is a horrible possibility, we are used to handling flammable materials and sometimes forget just how potentially dangerous they are. Some of the items under this heading are among those most often brought on to an aircraft accidentally. Avoid cigarette lighters and lighter fluid, devices powered by flammable materials (heaters, lamps etc.), flammable cleaning fluids, flammable gases (butane, methane, propane and other fuel gases), flammable paints and thinners, flammable solvents and adhesives, matches, paraffin (kerosene), petrol (gasoline). Safety matches and some types of lighter can be carried on the person only (they may accidentally rub against something in a bag). There is also a personal-care allowance of items like aerosols to take on, with limits of around 450 ml per item and 2 litres in total, but the best approach is to avoid these substances altogether.

appendix 6

Infectious materials

Few of us travel with medical specimens or bacterial or viral material in our baggage, but those for whom this is part of everyday work need to keep them off the plane.

Magnetic materials

An aircraft is filled with delicate instruments, some of which would not be very happy about the presence of a strong magnet. (Try putting a magnet up against an ordinary TV screen.) Avoid any strong magnets or equipment that may contain them, including large loudspeakers and specialist lab equipment.

Oxidizers

These are substances that encourage other things to burn or explode. They are essential components of explosives, and can encourage a spontaneous fire. Avoid bleach, chemical oxygen generators, fertilizers, fibreglass resin and repair kits, nitric acid, peroxides and specific oxidizing chemicals, and swimming-pool chemicals.

Poisons

The situation would not be good should these burst in the hold or generally get spread about the cabin. Specifically, any strong poison (including arsenic, cyanide etc.), insecticides (rather ironic, given that insecticide is sprayed on the passengers on some flights), pesticides, rodent killers and weed killers should not be carried.

Pressurized containers

This is an easy one to get wrong, as aerosol sprays and other pressurized cans are common household items that we rarely think of as dangerous. The can is designed to cope with the pressure difference between the inside and ordinary air pressure. But as the cabin pressure gets lower, particularly if there is any decompression, a pressurized container can explode like a small grenade. It's just not worth the risk. Specifically avoid aerosols (including deodorant, hair spray, insect repellent and spray paint), carbon-dioxide cartridges (often use for putting the fizz in fizzy drinks), oxygen tanks (for medical or diving purposes), self-defence sprays (Mace, pepper spray, tear gas etc.) and self-inflating devices such as life rafts.

Radioactive materials

Apart from the health risk for passengers, there is a danger that insufficiently shielded radioactive material may cause interference with the instrumentation and controls. Avoid radioactive products and medicines and the apparently innocuous smoke detectors.

Special materials

There are various hazardous materials that don't fit well into any of the other categories. Watch out for very cold materials that could react badly to low pressure or damage the aircraft (liquefied gases or dry ice, though some dry ice can be carried if appropriately vented).

Weapons

OK, most of us don't carry them anyway, except perhaps for sporting purposes, but if you live in a dangerous country you may be in the habit of keeping something about your person. On an aircraft this will not go down well. Specifically, avoid firearms (unloaded these can sometimes be carried in hold baggage, but check), knives (it's best to avoid even penknives), swords, throwing stars and other martial-arts weapons. Even sharp but apparently innocuous items like nail scissors and needles should only be placed in baggage going in the hold.

Appendix 7 Which Airline?

Each airline has a short code, used to identify it in flight numbers and other labels and signs. These two-way tables get you from code to airline or airline to code as quickly as possible.

Airline to code

Airline	Code	Airline	Code	Airline	Code
Aces Air	VX	Air Afrique	RK	Air Lanka Ltd	UL
Aer Lingus	EI	Air Belgium	AJ	Air Malta	KM
Aero California	JR	Air Canada	AC	Air New Zealand	NZ
Aero Peru	PL	Air China International	CA	Air Niugini	PX
Aeroflot Russian	SU	Air France	AF	Air Pacific	FJ
Aerolineas Argentinas	AR	Air India	AI	Air Zimbabwe	UM
Aeromexico	AM	Air Jamaica	JM	Alaska Airlines	AS

Airline	Code	Airline	Code	Airline	Code
Alitalia Airlines	AZ	Canadian Airlines	CP	Garuda Air	GA
All Nippon Airways	ANA	Cathay Pacific Airways	CX	Ghana Air	GH
Aloha Airlines	AQ	China Airlines	CI	Gulf Air Co.	GF
America Trans Air	TZ	China Eastern Air	MU	Hawaiian Airlines	HA
America West Airlines	HP	China Southern Airlines	CZ	Hong Kong Dragonair	KA
				Iberia Airlines	IB
American Airlines	AA	Continental Airlines	CO		
				Icelandair	FI
Ansett Airlines	AN	Continental Micronesia	CS		
				Japan Airlines	JL
AOM Airlines	IW	Copa Airlines	CM		
				Kenya Airways	KQ
Asiana Airlines	OZ	Czech Airlines	CSA		
				Kiwi International Air	KP
Austrian Airlines	OS	Delta Airlines	DL		
				KLM Royal Dutch Airlines	KL
Avianca	AV	Ecuatoriana	EU		
Aviateca	GU	Egypt Air	MS	Korean Airlines	KE
Balkan-Bulgarian	LZ	El Al Israel Airlines	LY	Kuwait Airways	KU
British Airways	BA	Emirates Air	EK	Lacsa Air	LR
British Midland	BD	Ethiopian Airlines	ET	Lan Chile Air	LA
BWIA International	BW	Eva Airways	BR	Lauda Air	NG
Cameroon Airlines	UY	Finnair	AY	Lloyd Aero Boliviano	LB

Airline	Code	Airline	Code	Airline	Code
Lot Polish	LO	Qantas Airways	QF	Tarom Romanian	RO
LTU International Airways	LT	Reno Air	QQ	Thai Airways International	TG
		Royal Air Maroc	AT		
Lufthansa Airlines	LU			Tower Air	FF
		Royal Jordanian	RJ		
Malaysia Airlines	MH			Trans Brasil Airlines	TR
		Royal Nepal Airlines	RA		
Malev Hungarian Airlines	MA			Trans World Airways	TW
		Sabena Airlines	SN		
				Transaero	UN
Mandarin Airlines	AE	Saeta Sociedad	EH	Turkish Airlines	TK
Martinair Holland	MP	Saudi Arabian Airlines	SV	Tyrolean	VO
Mexicana Airlines	MX	Scandinavian SAS	SK	United Airlines	UA
Middle East Airlines	ME	Singapore Airlines	SQ	US Airways	US
Namibia Air	SW	South African Air	SA	Varig Airlines	RG
Northwest Airlines	NW	Southwest Airlines	WN	Vasp Airlines	VP
Olympic Airlines	OA	Spanair	JK	Viasa	VA
Pakistan International	PK	Swissair	SR	Virgin Atlantic Airways	VS
Pan American Airlines	PA	Taca International	TA	World Airways	WO
Philippine Airlines	PR	TAP Air Portugal	TP	Yemen Airlines	IY

Code to airline

Code	Airline	Code	Airline	Code	Airline
AA	American Airlines	AZ	Alitalia Airlines	DL	Delta Airlines
AC	Air Canada	BA	British Airways	EH	Saeta Sociedad
AE	Mandarin Airlines	BD	British Midland	EI	Aer Lingus
AF	Air France	BR	Eva Airways	EK	Emirates Air
AI	Air India	BW	BWIA International	ET	Ethiopian Airlines
AJ	Air Belgium	CA	Air China International	EU	Ecuatoriana
AM	Aeromexico	CI	China Airlines	FF	Tower Air
AN	Ansett Airlines	CM	Copa Airlines	FI	Icelandair
ANA	All Nippon Airways	CO	Continental Airlines	FJ	Air Pacific
AQ	Aloha Airlines	CP	Canadian Airlines	GA	Garuda Air
AR	Aerolineas Argentinas	CS	Continental Micronesia	GF	Gulf Air Co.
AS	Alaska Airlines	CSA	Czech Airlines	GH	Ghana Air
AT	Royal Air Maroc	CX	Cathay Pacific Airways	GU	Aviateca
AV	Avianca	CZ	China Southern Airlines	HA	Hawaiian Airlines
AY	Finnair			HP	America West Airlines

Code	Airline	Code	Airline	Code	Airline
IB	Iberia Airlines	LR	Lacsa Air	OS	Austrian Airlines
IW	AOM Airlines	LT	LTU International Airways	OZ	Asiana Airlines
IY	Yemen Airlines			PA	Pan American Airlines
JK	Spanair	LU	Lufthansa Airlines	PK	Pakistan International
JL	Japan Airlines	LY	El Al Israel Airlines	PL	Aero Peru
JM	Air Jamaica	LZ	Balkan-Bulgarian	PR	Philippine Airlines
JR	Aero California	MA	Malev Hungarian Airlines	PX	Air Niugini
KA	Hong Kong Dragonair	ME	Middle East Airlines	QF	Qantas Airways
KE	Korean Airlines	MH	Malaysia Airlines	QQ	Reno Air
KL	KLM Royal Dutch Airlines	MP	Martinair Holland	RA	Royal Nepal Airlines
		MS	Egypt Air	RG	Varig Airlines
KM	Air Malta	MU	China Eastern Air	RJ	Royal Jordanian
KP	Kiwi International Air	MX	Mexicana Airlines	RK	Air Afrique
KQ	Kenya Airways	NG	Lauda Air	RO	Tarom Romanian
KU	Kuwait Airways	NW	Northwest Airlines	SA	South African Air
LA	Lan Chile Air	NZ	Air New Zealand	SK	Scandinavian SAS
LB	Lloyd Aero Boliviano	OA	Olympic Airlines	SN	Sabena Airlines
LO	Lot Polish	OK	Czech Airlines	SQ	Singapore Airlines

Code	Airline	Code	Airline	Code	Airline
SR	Swissair	TR	Trans Brasil Airlines	UY	Cameroon Airlines
SU	Aeroflot Russian	TW	Trans World Airways	VA	Viasa
SV	Saudi Arabian Airlines	TZ	America Trans Air	VO	Tyrolean
SW	Namibia Air	UA	United Airlines	VP	Vasp Airlines
TA	Taca International	UL	Air Lanka Ltd	VS	Virgin Atlantic Airways
TG	Thai Airways International	UM	Air Zimbabwe	VX	Aces Air
TK	Turkish Airlines	UN	Transaero	WN	Southwest Airlines
TP	TAP Air Portugal	US	US Airways	WO	World Airways

Appendix 8 Where Are we Going?

All airports have a three-letter code (known in the trade as a station code) by which they are known in airline computer systems. If you know the code of your destination airport you can make sure that you don't suffer lost bags as a result of a moment's lack of concentration by the check-in agent. A fair percentage of bags do get tagged with the wrong code – and go off on a magical mystery tour of their own.

The baggage tag has the airport code on it in large letters. Use this list to make a note of your destination codes. Don't assume that you will be able to guess them. They vary from the obvious (Manchester, UK, is MAN), via airport names (such as Paris, Charles de Gaulle, as CDG) to the downright obscure – like IAD for Dulles Airport at Washington, D.C., and a Y at the start of all the codes for Canadian cities. Note that codes beginning X are usually railway stations!

Code	Airport	Code	Airport
AAL	Aalborg, Denmark	AMD	Ahmadabad, India
AES	Aalesund, Norway (Vigra)	AJA	Ajaccio, France (Campo dell Oro)
AAR	Aarhus, Denmark (Tirstrup)	CAK	Akron/Canton, Ohio, USA
ABZ	Aberdeen, Scotland (Dyce)	AEY	Akureyri, Iceland
ABR	Aberdeen, S. Dak., USA	ALM	Alamogordo, N. Mex., USA
ABJ	Abidjan, Ivory Coast (Port Bouet)	ALS	Alamosa, Colo., USA (Bergman Field)
ABI	Abilene, Tex., USA	ABY	Albany G., USA (Dougherty County)
AUH	Abu Dhabi, United Arab Emirates	ALB	Albany, N.Y., USA
ABS	Abu Simbel, Egypt	ABQ	Albuquerque, N. Mex., USA
ACA	Acapulco, Mexico (Alvarez)	ABX	Albury, N.S.W., Australia
ACC	Accra, Ghana (Kotoka)	ACI	Alderney, Channel Islands (The Blaye)
ADA	Adana, Turkey	ALP	Aleppo, Syria (Nejrab)
ADD	Addis Ababa, Ethiopia (Bole)	ALY	Alexandria, Egypt
ADL	Adelaide, S.A., Australia	AEX	Alexandria, La., USA
AGA	Agadir, Morocco (Inezgane)	XFS	Alexandria, Ont., Canada
AGF	Agen, France (La Garenne)	AXD	Alexandroupolis, Greece
AGR	Agra, India (Kheria)	AHO	Alghero, Italy (Fertilia)
BQN	Aguadilla, P.R., USA		
AGU	Aguascalientes, Mexico		

Code	Airport	Code	Airport
ALG	Algiers, Algeria (Houari Boumédienne)	ADJ	Amman, Jordan (Civil)
ALC	Alicante, Spain	AMM	Amman, Jordan (Queen Alia International)
ASP	Alice Springs, N.T., Australia	YEY	Amos, Que., Canada
AET	Allakaket, Alaska, USA	AMS	Amsterdam, Netherlands (Schipol)
ABE	Allentown, Pa., USA	ANC	Anchorage, Alaska, USA
AIA	Alliance, Nebr., USA	AOI	Ancona, Italy (Falconara)
ALA	Almaty, Kazakhstan	ASD	Andros Town, Bahamas
LEI	Almeíra, Spain	ANG	Angoulême, France (Gel-Air)
AOR	Alor Setar, Malaysia (Sultan Abdul Halim)	AXA	Anguilla
GUR	Alotau, Papua New Guinea (Gurney)	ANI	Aniak, Alaska, USA
APN	Alpena, Mich., USA	AJN	Anjouan, Comoros
ALE	Alpine, Tex., USA	ESB	Ankara, Turkey (Esenboga)
ALF	Alta, Norway (Elvebakken)	AAE	Annaba, Algeria (Les Salines)
AOO	Altoona/Martinsburg, Pa., USA (Blair County)	NCY	Annecy, France (Annecy-Meythe)
		ANB	Anniston, Ala., USA
AMA	Amarillo, Tex., USA	AYT	Antalya, Turkey
ABL	Ambler, Alaska, USA	TNR	Antananarivo, Madagascar (Ivato)
AMQ	Ambon, Indonesia (Pattimura)	ANF	Antofagasta, Chile (Cerro Moreno)

Code	Airport
ANR	Antwerp, Belgium (Deurne)
ANV	Anvik, Alaska, USA
AOJ	Aomori, Japan
APW	Apia, Samoa (Faleolo)
ATW	Appleton, Wis., USA (Outagamie County)
AQJ	Aqaba, Jordan
AJU	Aracaju, Sergipe, Brazil
AUC	Arauca, Colombia
ACV	Arcata Calif., USA (Arcata/Eureka)
AQP	Arequipa, Peru (Rodriguez Ballon)
ARI	Arica, Chile (Chacalluta)
ARH	Arkhangelsk, Russia
ARM	Armidale, N.S.W., Australia
ATC	Arthur's Town, Bahamas
AUA	Aruba (Reina Beatrix)
AKJ	Asahikawa, Japan
AVL	Asheville/Hendersonville, N.C., USA
ASM	Asmara, Eritrea

Code	Airport
ASE	Aspen, Colo., USA (Pitkin County/ Sardy Field)
OVD	Asturias, Spain
ASU	Asunción, Paraguay (Silvio Pettirossi)
ASW	Aswan, Egypt (Daraw)
AHN	Athens, Ga., USA
ATH	Athens, Greece (Hellinikon)
YIB	Atikokan, Ont., Canada
ATL	Atlanta, Ga., USA (Hartsfield International)
ACY	Atlantic City, N.J., USA
AKL	Auckland, New Zealand
AGB	Augsburg, Germany (Muehlhausen)
AGS	Augusta, Ga., USA (Bush Field)
AUG	Augusta, Maine, USA (Maine State)
IXU	Aurangabad, India (Chikkalthana)
AUS	Austin, Tex., USA (Robert Mueller Municipal)
AVN	Avignon, France (Caumont)

Code	Airport	Code	Airport
AYQ	Ayers Rock, N.T., Australia (Connellan)	BGR	Bangor, Maine, USA
		BGF	Bangui, Central African Republic
BCD	Bacolod, Philippines	BDJ	Banjarmasin, Indonesia (Syamsudin Noor)
IXB	Bagdogra, India		
BHI	Bahía Blanca, Argentina (Commandante)	BJL	Banjul, Gambia (Yundum International)
BAH	Bahrain	BHB	Bar Harbor, Maine, USA
YBC	Baie Comeau, Que., Canada	BCN	Barcelona, Spain
BFL	Bakersfield, Calif., USA (Meadows Field)	BLA	Barcelona, Venezuela
		BRI	Bari, Italy
BAK	Baku, Azerbaijan	BNS	Barinas, Venezuela
BWI	Baltimore, Md., USA	BAX	Barnaul, Russia
ABM	Bamaga, Qld., Australia	BRM	Barquisimeto, Venezuela
BKO	Bamako, Mali (Senou)	BRR	Barra, Hebrides, Scotland (Northay)
BWN	Bandar Seri Begawan, Brunei	EJA	Barrancabermeja, Colombia (Variguies)
BDO	Bandung, Indonesia (Husein Sastranegara)	BAQ	Barranquilla, Colombia (E. Cortissoz)
YBA	Banff, Alta., Canada	BRW	Barrow, Alaska, USA
BLR	Bangalore, India (Hindustan)	BSL	Basel, Switzerland
BKK	Bangkok, Thailand	EAP	Basel/Mulhouse Switzerland/France

Code	Airport
BIA	Bastia, Corsica (Poretta)
BHS	Bathurst, N.S.W., Australia (Raglan)
BRT	Bathurst Island, N.T., Australia
BAL	Batman, Turkey
BYU	Bayreuth, Germany (Bindlacher Berg)
BPT	Beaumont, Tex., USA (Jefferson County)
BKW	Beckley, W.Va., USA
BED	Bedford, Mass., USA
BEI	Beica, Ethiopia
NAY	Beijing, China
PEK	Beijing, China (Peking Capital Airport)
BEW	Beira, Mozambique
BEY	Beirut, Lebanon
BEL	Belém, Brazil (Val de Cans)
BHD	Belfast, Northern Ireland (Belfast Harbour)

Code	Airport
BFS	Belfast, Northern Ireland (International)
BEG	Belgrade, Serbia
BZE	Belize City, Belize (International)
TZA	Belize City, Belize (Municipal)
XVV	Belleville, Ont., Canada
BLI	Bellingham, Wash., USA
PLU	Belo Horizonte, Brazil (Confins/Pampulha)
CNF	Belo Horizonte, Brazil (Tancredo Neves)
BJI	Bemidji, Minn., USA
BEH	Benton Harbor, Mich., USA (Ross Field)
BGO	Bergen, Norway (Flesland)
BER	Berlin, Germany (Schönefeld)
SXF	Berlin, Germany (Schönefeld)
TXL	Berlin, Germany (Tegel)
THF	Berlin, Germany (Tempelhof)

Code	Airport
BDA	Bermuda (Kindley Airfield/Civil Air Terminal)
BRN	Berne, Switzerland (Belp)
BZR	Béziers, France (Béziers-Vias)
ZDJ	Berne, Switzerland (Berne-Railway Station)
BET	Bethel, Alaska, USA
BWA	Bhairawa, Nepal
BBI	Bhubaneswar, India
BIK	Biak, Indonesia (Mokmer)
BIQ	Biarritz, France (Parme)
BGK	Big Creek, Belize
BIO	Bilbao, Spain (Sondica)
BIL	Billings, Mont., USA
BLL	Billund, Denmark
BIM	Bimini, Bahamas (International)
NSB	Bimini, Bahamas (North Seaplane Base)
BGM	Binghamton/Endicott/Johnson City, N.Y., USA

Code	Airport
BTU	Bintulu, Sarawak, Malaysia
BVI	Birdsville, Qld., Australia
BHM	Birmingham, Ala., USA (Seibels/Bryan)
BHX	Birmingham, England
FRU	Bishkek, Kyrgyzstan
BSK	Biskra, Algeria
BIS	Bismarck, N.Dak., USA
OXB	Bissau, Guinea-Bissau (Osvaldo Vieira)
BLK	Blackpool, England
YBZ	Blanc Sablon, Que., Canada
BLZ	Blantyre, Malawi (Chileka)
BFN	Bloemfontein, South Africa (JBM Hertzog)
BMI	Bloomington, Ill., USA (Normal)
BMG	Bloomington, Ind., USA (Monroe County)
BLF	Bluefield, W.Va., USA
BVB	Boa Vista, Roraima, Brazil

Code	Airport	Code	Airport
BOO	Bodo, Norway	XPN	Brampton, Ont., Canada
BXN	Bodrum, Turkey (Imsik)	YBR	Brandon, Man., Canada
BOG	Bogotá, Colombia (Eldorado)	XFV	Brantford, Ont., Canada
BOI	Boise, Idaho, USA (Gowen Field)	BSB	Brasília, Distrito Federal, Brazil
BLQ	Bologna, Italy (Guglielmo Marconi)	BTS	Bratislava, Slovakia (Ivanka)
BOM	Bombay, India	QKB	Breckenridge Colo., USA
BON	Bonaire, Netherlands Antilles (Flamingo Field)	BRE	Bremen, Germany
		PWT	Bremerton, Wash., USA
YVB	Bonaventure, Que., Canada	BES	Brest, France (Guipavas)
BNJ	Bonn, Germany	BDR	Bridgeport, Conn., USA (Sikorsky Memorial)
BOD	Bordeaux, France (Merignac)		
RNN	Bornholm, Denmark (Arnager)	BGI	Bridgetown, Barbados (Grantley Adams)
BOS	Boston, Mass., USA (Logan International)	BNE	Brisbane, Qld., Australia
WBU	Boulder, Colo., USA	BRS	Bristol, England
BZN	Bozeman, Mont., USA (Gallatin Field)	TRI	Bristol/Johnson City/Kingsport, Tenn., USA
LBA	Bradford, England	BVE	Brive-La-Gaillarde, France (Laroche)
BFD	Bradford, Pa., USA	BRQ	Brno, Czech Republic (Turany)
BRD	Brainerd, Minn., USA	XBR	Brockville, Ont., Canada

Code	Airport
BHQ	Broken Hill, N.S.W., Australia
BNN	Bronnoysund, Norway
BKX	Brookings, S.Dak., USA
BRO	Brownsville, Tex., USA (South Padre Island)
BQK	Brunswick, Ga., USA (Glynco Jetport)
BRU	Brussels, Belgium
BGA	Bucaramanga, Colombia (Palo Negro)
BBU	Bucharest, Romania (Băneasa)
OTP	Bucharest, Romania (Otopeni)
BUD	Budapest, Hungary (Ferihegy)
EZE	Buenos Aires, Argentina (Eze)
AEP	Buenos Aires, Argentina (Jorge Newberry)
BUF	Buffalo, N.Y., USA
BHK	Bukhara, Uzbekistan
BUQ	Bulawayo, Zimbabwe
IFP	Bullhead City, Ariz., USA

Code	Airport
BUR	Burbank, Calif., USA
BRL	Burlington, Iowa, USA
BTV	Burlington, V., USA
YPZ	Burns Lake, B.C., Canada
BUZ	Bushehr, Iran
BTM	Butte, Mont., USA
BXU	Butuan, Philippines
CFR	Caen, France (Carpiquet)
CAG	Cagliari, Sardinia, Italy (Elmas)
CNS	Cairns, Qld., Australia
CAI	Cairo, Egypt
CCU	Calcutta, India
YYC	Calgary, Alberta, Canada
CLO	Cali, Colombia (Alfonso Bonilla Aragon)
CCJ	Calicut, India
CLY	Calvi, Corsica, France (Ste Catherine)
CBG	Cambridge, England

Code	Airport
CDH	Camden, Ark., USA
YBL	Campbell River, B.C., Canada
XAZ	Campbellton, N.B., Canada
CPQ	Campinas, São Paulo, Brazil
CGR	Campo Grande, Mato Grosso do Sul, Brazil
CAJ	Canaima, Venezuela
CBR	Canberra, Australia
CUN	Cancún, Mexico
JCA	Cannes, France (Mandelieu)
CGI	Cape Girardeau, Mo., USA
CPT	Cape Town, South Africa (D. F. Malan)
XAW	Capreol, Ont., Canada
CCS	Caracas, Venezuela (Simon Bolívar)
CKS	Carajás, Pará, Brazil
MDH	Carbondale, Ill., USA
CCF	Carcassonne, France (Salvaza)
CWL	Cardiff, Wales

Code	Airport
CLD	Carlsbad, Calif., USA (Carlsbad/ Palomar)
CRU	Carriacou Island, Grenada
CTG	Cartagena, Colombia (Rafael Núñez)
CUP	Carúpano, Venezuela
LRM	Casa de Campo, Dominican Republic
CAS	Casablanca, Morocco (Anfa)
CMN	Casablanca, Morocco (Mohamed V)
CPR	Casper, Wyo., USA (Natrona County)
XZB	Casselman, Ont., Canada
YCG	Castlegar, B.C., Canada
CTA	Catania, Sicily, Italy (Fontanarossa)
CAY	Cayenne, French Guiana (Rochambeau)
CYB	Cayman Brac Island, Cayman Islands
CEB	Cebu, Philippines
CDC	Cedar City, Utah, USA
CID	Cedar Rapids, Iowa, USA
CDR	Chadron, Nebr., USA

Code	Airport	Code	Airport
CMF	Chambéry, France (Chambéry/Aix-les-Bains)	CHA	Chattanooga, Tenn., USA (Charles Lovell Field)
XCI	Chambord, Que., Canada	CJU	Cheju, South Korea
CMI	Champaign, Ill., USA (Univ. of Illinois–Willard)	XHS	Chemainus, B.C., Canada
		CTU	Chengdu, China
XDL	Chandler, Que., Canada	CER	Cherbourg, France (Maupertus)
CGQ	Changchun, China	CYS	Cheyenne, Wyo., USA
CSX	Changsha, China	CNX	Chiang Mai, Thailand
CHQ	Chania, Crete, Greece (Souda)	CEI	Chiang Rai, Thailand
YLD	Chapleau, Ont., Canada	YMT	Chibougamau, Que., Canada
CHS	Charleston, SC., USA	CGX	Chicago, Ill., USA (Meigs Field)
CRW	Charleston, W.Va., USA (Yeager)	MDW	Chicago, Ill., USA (Midway)
CTL	Charleville, Qld., Australia	ORD	Chicago, Ill., USA (O'Hare)
CLT	Charlotte, N.C., USA (Charlotte/Douglas)	PWK	Chicago, Ill., USA (Pal-Waukee)
		CIX	Chiclayo, Peru (Cornel Ruiz)
CHO	Charlottesville, Va., USA (Charlottesville/Albemarle)	CIC	Chico, Calif., USA
		KCG	Chignik, Alaska, USA (Fisheries)
YYG	Charlottetown, P.E.I., Canada	KCL	Chignik, Alaska, USA (Lagoon)
XCM	Chatham, Ont., Canada	CUU	Chihuahua, Mexico (Gen. Villa-Lobos)

Code	Airport	Code	Airport
CGP	Chittagong, Bangladesh (Patenga)	CLL	College Station, Tex., USA
CHC	Christchurch, New Zealand	QKL	Cologne, Germany (Railway Station)
YYQ	Churchill, Manitoba, Canada	CGN	Cologne/Bonn, Germany (Köln/Bonn)
CVG	Cincinnati, Ohio, USA	CMB	Colombo, Sri Lanka (Katunayake)
CBL	Ciudad Bolívar, Venezuela	CYR	Colonia, Uruguay
CME	Ciudad del Carmen, Campeche, Mexico	COS	Colorado Springs, Colo., USA
		COU	Columbia, Mo., USA
CJS	Ciudad Juárez, Chihuahua, Mexico	CAE	Columbia, S.C., USA
CEN	Ciudad Obregón, Sonora, Mexico	CSG	Columbus, Ga., USA (Columbus/Fort Benning)
CKB	Clarksburg, W.Va., USA (Clarksburg-Benedum)		
		GTR	Columbus, Miss., USA (Golden)
CLE	Cleveland, Ohio, USA (Hopkins)	CMH	Columbus, Ohio, USA (Port Columbus)
CVN	Clovis, N. Mex., USA		
CLJ	Cluj, Romania	CRD	Comodoro Rivadavia, Chubut, Argentina
XGJ	Cobourg, Ont., Canada		
CBB	Cochabamba, Bolivia (San José de la Banda)	YQQ	Comox, B.C., Canada
		CKY	Conakry, Guinea
COK	Cochin, India (Naval Air Station)	CCP	Concepción, Chile (Carriel Sur)
CJB	Coimbatore, India (Peelamedu)	NOC	Connaught, Ireland
CLQ	Colima, Mexico	CND	Constanţa, Romania (Kogălniceanu)

Code	Airport	Code	Airport
OOM	Cooma, N.S.W., Australia	YXC	Cranbrook, B.C., Canada
CPH	Copenhagen, Denmark	CEC	Crescent City, Calif., USA
YCO	Coppermine, N.W.T., Canada	CRI	Crooked Island, Bahamas
COR	Córdoba, Argentina (Pajas Blancas)	CUC	Cúcuta, Colombia (Camilo Daza)
CDV	Cordova, Alaska, USA	CUE	Cuenca, Ecuador (Mariscal la Mar)
ORK	Cork, Ireland	CGB	Cuiabá, Mato Grosso, Brazil
YCC	Cornwall, Ont., Canada	CUL	Culiacan, Sinaloa, Mexico
CRP	Corpus Christi, Tex., USA	CUM	Cumana, Venezuela
CEZ	Cortez, Colo., USA (Montezuma County)	CBE	Cumberland, Md., USA
CMG	Corumbá, Mato Grosso do Sul, Brazil	CWB	Curitiba, Paraná, Brazil (Afonso Peña)
XGK	Coteau, Que., Canada	CUZ	Cuzco, Peru (Velazco Astete)
COO	Cotonou, Benin	DAD	Da Nang, Vietnam
KIR	County Kerry, Ireland	DKR	Dakar, Senegal (Yoff)
YCA	Courtenay, B.C., Canada	DLM	Dalaman, Turkey
CWT	Cowra, N.S.W., Australia	DLC	Dalian, China
GXQ	Coyhaique, Chile (Teniente Vidal)	DAL	Dallas, Tex., USA (Love Field)
CZM	Cozumel, Quintana Roo, Mexico	DFW	Dallas/Fort Worth, Tex., USA
CGA	Craig, Alaska, USA	DAM	Damascus, Syria

Code	Airport
DGA	Dangriga, Belize
DNV	Danville, Ill., USA (Vermilion County)
DAN	Danville, Va., USA
DAR	Dar es Salaam, Tanzania
DRW	Darwin, N.T., Australia
YDN	Dauphin, Man., Canada
DVO	Davao, Philippines (Mati)
YDQ	Dawson Creek, B.C., Canada
DAY	Dayton, Ohio, USA (James M. Cox)
DAB	Daytona Beach, Fla., USA
LGI	Deadmans Cay/Long Island, Bahamas
DOL	Deauville, France (Saint Gatien)
DEC	Decatur, Ill., USA
YDF	Deer Lake, Nfld., Canada
YVZ	Deer Lake, Ont., Canada
DRT	Del Rio, Tex., USA
DEL	Delhi, India
DEM	Dembidollo, Ethiopia

Code	Airport
DNM	Denham, W.A., Australia
DPS	Denpasar Bali, Indonesia (Ngurah Rai)
DEN	Denver, Colo., USA
DSM	Des Moines, Iowa, USA
DSI	Destin, Fla., USA
DTW	Detroit, Mich., USA
DPO	Devonport, Tas., Australia
DHA	Dhahran, Saudi Arabia
DAC	Dhaka, Bangladesh (Zia International)
DIB	Dibrugarh, India (Chabua)
DIJ	Dijon, France (Longvic)
DIL	Dili, Indonesia (Comoro)
DPL	Dipolog, Philippines
DIY	Diyarbakir, Turkey
JIB	Djibouti, Djibouti (Ambouli)
DDC	Dodge City, Kans., USA
DOH	Doha, Qatar

Code	Airport
DCF	Dominica, Dominica (Cane Field)
DOM	Dominica, Dominica (Melville Hal-Dom)
DOK	Donetsk, Ukraine
DTM	Dortmund, Germany (Wickede)
DHN	Dothan, Ala., USA
DLA	Douala, Cameroon
DRS	Dresden, Germany
XDM	Drummondville, Que., Canada
YHD	Dryden, Ont., Canada
DUJ	Du Bois, Pa., USA (Jefferson County)
DXB	Dubai, United Arab Emirates
DBO	Dubbo, N.S.W., Australia
DUB	Dublin, Ireland
DBQ	Dubuque, Iowa, USA
DLH	Duluth, Minn., USA
DUQ	Duncan/Quam, B.C., Canada
DND	Dundee, Scotland

Code	Airport
DUD	Dunedin, New Zealand (Momona)
DRO	Durango, Colo., USA (Durango La Plata)
DGO	Durango, Mexico (Gen. Guadalupe Victoria)
DUR	Durban, South Africa (Louis Botha)
DUS	Düsseldorf, Germany
QDU	Düsseldorf, Germany (Main Station)
DUT	Dutch Harbor, Alaska, USA
ELS	East London, South Africa (Ben Shoeman)
EMA	East Midlands, England
IPC	Easter Island, Chile (Mataveri)
ESD	Eastsound, Wash., USA
EAU	Eau Claire Wis., USA
EDI	Edinburgh, Scotland (Turnhouse)
YEG	Edmonton, Alta., Canada (International)
YXD	Edmonton, Alta, Canada (Municipal)
EDR	Edward River, Qld., Australia

Code	Airport	Code	Airport
ETH	Eilat, Israel	EBJ	Esbjerg, Denmark
EIN	Eindhoven, Netherlands (Welschap)	ESC	Escanaba, Mich., USA (Delta County)
SVX	Ekaterinburg, Russia	EPR	Esperance, W.A., Australia
ELD	El Dorado, Ark., USA	YPF	Esquimalt, B.C., Canada
ELP	El Paso, Tex., USA	EUG	Eugene, Oreg., USA
ESR	El Salvador, Chile	EVV	Evansville, Ind., USA
EBA	Elba Island, Italy (Marina di Campo)	EVE	Evenes, Norway
EKO	Elko, Nev., USA (J. C. Harris Field)	EXE	Exeter, England
YEL	Elliot Lake, Ont., Canada	FAE	Faeroe Islands
ELM	Elmira/Corning, N.Y., USA	FAI	Fairbanks, Alaska, USA
ELY	Ely, Nev., USA (Yelland Field)	FRM	Fairmont, Minn., USA
EMD	Emerald, Qld., Australia	LYP	Faisalabad, Pakistan (Lyallpur)
WDG	Enid, Okla., USA (Woodring Municipal)	FAR	Fargo, N.Dak., USA (Hector Airport)
ENS	Enschede, Netherlands (Twente)	FMN	Farmington, N. Mex., USA (Four Corners)
EBB	Entebbe/Kampala, Uganda	FAO	Faro, Portugal
ERF	Erfurt, Germany	FYV	Fayetteville, Ark., USA
ERI	Erie, Pa., USA	FAY	Fayetteville, N.C., USA
ERZ	Erzurum, Turkey	FFM	Fergus Falls, Minn., USA

Code	Airport	Code	Airport
FEZ	Fez, Morocco	RSW	Fort Myers, Fla., USA (Regional Southwest)
FLG	Flagstaff, Ariz., USA		
FNT	Flint, Mich., USA (Bishop)	YXJ	Fort St John, B.C., Canada
FLR	Florence, Italy	YFS	Fort Simpson, N.W.T., Canada
FLO	Florence, S.C., USA (Gilbert Field)	FSM	Fort Smith, Ark., USA
FRS	Flores, Guatemala	YSM	Fort Smith, N.W.T., Canada
FLN	Florianopolis, Santa Catarina, Brazil	FWA	Fort Wayne, Ind., USA (Baer Field)
FRO	Florø, Norway	FOR	Fortaleza, Ceará, Brazil
FDE	Forde, Norway	FRA	Frankfurt am Main, Germany
FMA	Formosa, Argentina	FKL	Franklin, Pa., USA (Chess Lamberton)
FNL	Fort Collins/Loveland, Colo., USA		
FDF	Fort de France, Martinique	YFC	Fredericton, N.B., Canada
FOD	Fort Dodge, Iowa, USA	FPO	Freeport, Bahamas
FHU	Fort Huachuca/Sierra Vista, Ariz., USA	FAT	Fresno, Calif., USA (Fresno Air Terminal)
FLL	Fort Lauderdale, Fla., USA (Ft Lauderdale/Hollywood)	FRD	Friday Harbor, Wash., USA
		FDH	Friedrichshafen, Germany (Friedrichshafen/Lowenthal)
TBN	Fort Leonard Wood, Mo., USA (Forney Field)		
		FUE	Fuerteventura/Puerto del Rosario, Canary Islands, Spain
YMM	Fort McMurray, Alta., Canada		

Code	Airport
FUK	Fukuoka, Japan (Itazuke)
FNC	Funchal, Madeira, Portugal
GBE	Gaborone, Botswana
GNV	Gainesville, Fla., USA (Jr Alison Municipal)
GPS	Galapagos Islands, Ecuador (Baltra)
GAL	Galena, Alaska, USA
GBG	Galesburg, Ill., USA
GUP	Gallup N. Mex., USA
GLS	Galveston, Tex., USA (Scholes Field)
GWY	Galway, Ireland (Carnmore)
YQX	Gander, Nfld., Canada
GCK	Garden City, Kans., USA
GYY	Gary, Ind., USA
YGP	Gaspe, Que., Canada
YND	Gatineau, Que., Canada
GAU	Gauhati, India (Borjhar)
GDN	Gdańsk, Poland (Rebiechowo)
GVA	Geneva, Switzerland

Code	Airport
GOA	Genoa, Italy (Christoforo Colombo)
GRJ	George, South Africa
GGT	George Town, Bahamas (Exuma)
GEO	Georgetown, Guyana (Timehri)
XHM	Georgetown, Ont., Canada
GET	Geraldton, W.A., Australia
GRO	Gerona, Spain (Costa Brava)
GIB	Gibraltar, Gibraltar
YGX	Gillam, Man., Canada
GCC	Gillette, Wyo., USA (Campbell County)
YGB	Gillies Bay, B.C., Canada
GGW	Glasgow, Mont., USA
GLA	Glasgow, Scotland
PIK	Glasgow, Scotland (Prestwick)
XZC	Glencoe, Ont., Canada
GDV	Glendive, Mont., USA
GOI	Goa, India (Dabolim)
ZGI	Gods River, Man., Canada

Code	Airport
OOL	Gold Coast, Qld., Australia (Coolangatta)
GLF	Golfito, Costa Rica
GLV	Golovin, Alaska, USA
GLD	Goodland, Kans., USA (Renner Field)
YYR	Goose Bay, Nfld, Canada
GKA	Goroka, Papua New Guinea
GTO	Gorontalo, Indonesia (Tolotio)
GOT	Gothenburg, Sweden (Landvetter)
GOV	Gove, N.T., Australia (Nhulunbuy)
GHB	Governor's Harbour, Bahamas
LPA	Gran Canaria, Canary Islands, Spain
GRX	Granada, Spain
GCN	Grand Canyon, Ariz., USA
GCM	Grand Cayman, Cayman Islands (Owen Roberts)
GFK	Grand Forks, N.Dak., USA
GRI	Grand Island, Nebr., USA (Central Nebraska)

Code	Airport
GJT	Grand Junction, Colo., USA (Walker Field)
GRR	Grand Rapids, Mich., USA (Kent County)
GDT	Grand Turk Island, Turks and Caicos
YQU	Grande Prairie, Alta., Canada
GRZ	Graz, Austria (Thalerhof)
GTF	Great Falls, Mont., USA
GRB	Green Bay, Wis., USA (Austin/Straybel)
LWB	Greenbrier W.Va., USA
GSO	Greensboro/High Point, N.C., USA (Piedmont)
PGV	Greenville, N.C., USA
GNB	Grenoble, France (St-Geoirs)
XGY	Grimsby, Ont., Canada
GRQ	Groningen, Netherlands (Eelde)
GON	Groton/New London, Conn., USA
GDL	Guadalajara, Mexico (Miguel Hidalgo)
GUM	Guam, Guam (Ab Wonpat)

Code	Airport
CAN	Guangzhou, China (Baiyun)
GUA	Guatemala City, Guatemala (La Aurora)
GYE	Guayaquil, Ecuador (Simon Bolivar)
GYM	Guaymas, Sonora, Mexico
XIA	Guelph, Ont., Canada
GCI	Guernsey, Channel Islands
GUB	Guerrero Negro, Baja California Sur, Mexico
KWL	Guilin, China
GPT	Gulfport, Miss., USA (Gulfport/Biloxi)
GUC	Gunnison, Colo., USA
GWD	Gwadar, Pakistan
HGR	Hagerstown, Md., USA (Washington County)
HAK	Haikou, China
HNS	Haines, Alaska, USA
HKD	Hakodate, Japan
YHZ	Halifax, N.S., Canada
HAD	Halmstad, Sweden

Code	Airport
HAM	Hamburg, Germany (Fuhlsbuttel)
HLZ	Hamilton, New Zealand (Hamilton)
YHM	Hamilton, Ontario, Canada
HTI	Hamilton Island, Qld., Australia
HFT	Hammerfest, Norway
CMX	Hancock, Mich., USA (Houghton County)
HGH	Hangzhou, China
HAN	Hanoi, Vietnam (Noibai)
HAJ	Hanover, Germany (Langenhagen)
HRE	Harare, Zimbabwe
HRB	Harbin, China
HRL	Harlingen, Tex., USA
MDT	Harrisburg, Pa., USA
HRO	Harrison, Ark., USA (Boone County)
BDL	Hartford, Conn., USA (Bradley International)
HSI	Hastings, Nebr., USA
HDY	Hat Yai, Thailand

Code	Airport	Code	Airport
HAU	Haugesund, Norway (Karmoy)	HKY	Hickory, N.C., USA
HAV	Havana, Cuba (José Marti)	YOJ	High Level, Alta., Canada (Footner Lake)
HVR	Havre, Mont., USA (City County)		
YHY	Hay River, N.W.T., Canada	ITO	Hilo, Hawaii, USA (Hawaii International)
HDN	Hayden, Colo., USA (Yampa Valley)	HHH	Hilton Head, S.C., USA
HIS	Hayman Island, Qld., Australia	HIJ	Hiroshima, Japan
HYS	Hays, Kans., USA	SGN	Ho Chi Minh City, Vietnam (Tan Son Nhut)
HDB	Heidelberg, Germany		
HLN	Helena, Mont., USA	HBA	Hobart, Tas., Australia
AGH	Helsingborg, Sweden (Angelholm/ Helsingborg)	HOB	Hobbs, N. Mex., USA (Lea County)
		HET	Hohhot, China
JHE	Helsingborg, Sweden (Heliport)	HKK	Hokitika, New Zealand
HEL	Helsinki, Finland	YHI	Holman Island, N.W.T., Canada
HER	Heraklion, Crete, Greece	HOM	Homer, Alaska, USA
HMO	Hermosillo, Mexico (Gen. Ignacio Garcia)	HJK	Hong Kong
		HIR	Honiara/Guadalcanal, Solomon Islands
XDU	Hervey, Quebec, Canada		
HVB	Hervey Bay, Qld., Australia	HNL	Honolulu, Hawaii, USA
HIB	Hibbing/Chisholm, Minn., USA	MKK	Hoolehua, Hawaii, USA

Code	Airport	Code	Airport
HNH	Hoonah, Alaska, USA	HRG	Hurghada, Egypt
HPB	Hooper Bay, Alaska, USA	HON	Huron, S.Dak., USA
YHN	Hornepayne, Ont., Canada	HWN	Hwange National Park, Zimbabwe
HKN	Hoskins, Papua New Guinea	HYA	Hyannis, Mass., USA (Barnstable County)
HOT	Hot Springs, Ark., USA (Memorial Field)		
		HYG	Hydaburg, Alaska, USA
HUM	Houma, La., USA (Terrebonne)	HYD	Hyderabad, India (Begumpet)
ZHO	Houston, B.C., Canada	IAS	Iaşi, Romania
EFD	Houston, Tex., USA (Ellington Field)	IBZ	Ibiza, Spain
HOU	Houston, Tex., USA (Houston Hobby)	IDA	Idaho Falls, Idaho, USA
IAH	Houston, Tex., USA (Intercontinental)	YGT	Igloolik, N.W.T., Canada
HUN	Hualien, Taiwan	IGU	Iguaçu Falls, Paraná, Brazil
HUX	Huatulco, Oaxaca, Mexico	IGR	Iguazu, Misiones, Argentina
YHB	Hudson Bay, Sask., Canada	YGR	Îles de la Madeleine, Que., Canada
HUI	Hue, Vietnam	ILF	Ilford, Man., Canada
HUY	Humberside, England	IOS	Ilhéus, Bahía, Brazil (Eduardo Gómes)
HTS	Huntington/Ashland, W.Va., USA (Tri-State)		
		ILI	Iliamna, Alaska, USA
HSV	Huntsville/Decatur, Ala., USA (Madison County)	ILQ	Ilo, Moquegua, Peru

Code	Airport
ILO	Iloilo, Philippines (Mandurriao)
JAV	Ilulissat, Greenland
IMP	Imperatriz, Maranhão, Brazil
IMF	Imphal, India
IGA	Inagua, Bahamas
SHC	Indaselassie, Ethiopia
IND	Indianapolis, Ind., USA
XIB	Ingersoll, Ont., Canada
INN	Innsbruck, Austria (Kranebitten)
INL	International Falls, Minn., USA
YEV	Inuvik, N.W.T., Canada
INV	Inverness, Scotland
IYK	Inyokern, Calif., USA
IOA	Ioannina, Greece
IPI	Ipiales, Colombia (San Luis)
YFB	Iqaluit, N.W.T., Canada
IQQ	Iquique, Chile (Chucumata)
IQT	Iquitos, Peru (cf. Secada)
IKT	Irkutsk, Russia

Code	Airport
IMT	Iron Mountain, Mich., USA (Ford)
IWD	Ironwood, Mich., USA (Gogebic County)
ISB	Islamabad, Pakistan
ILY	Islay, Scotland (Glenegedale)
IOM	Isle of Man, United Kingdom (Ronaldsway)
ISC	Isles of Scilly, United Kingdom (Tresco)
ISP	Islip, N.Y., USA (Long Island–Macarthur)
IST	Istanbul, Turkey (Atatürk)
ITH	Ithaca, N.Y., USA (Tompkins County)
ZIH	Ixtapa/Zihuatanejo, Guerrero, Mexico
IJK	Izhevsk, Russia
ADB	Izmir, Turkey (Adnam Menderes)
IZO	Izumo, Japan
JAT	Jabat, Marshall Islands
JAN	Jackson, Miss., USA (Allen C. Thompson Field)

Code	Airport	Code	Airport
MKL	Jackson, Tenn., USA (McKellar Field)	JNB	Johannesburg, South Africa (Jan Smuts)
JAC	Jackson Hole, Wyo., USA	JON	Johnston Island, USA, Outlying Islands
JAX	Jacksonville, Fla., USA		
OAJ	Jacksonville, N.C., USA	JST	Johnstown, Pa., USA
JAI	Jaipur, India (Sanganeer)	JHB	Johor Baharu, Malaysia (Sultan Ismail)
HLP	Jakarta, Indonesia (Halim Perdana Kusama)	JOI	Joinville, Santa Catarina, Brazil
		XJL	Joliette, Que., Canada
CGK	Jakarta, Indonesia (Sukarno-Hatta)	JMO	Jomsom, Nepal
JMS	Jamestown, N.Dak., USA	JBR	Jonesboro, Ark., USA
JHW	Jamestown, N.Y., USA (Chautauqua County)	JKG	Jönköping, Sweden (Axamo)
IXJ	Jammu, India (Satwari)	XJQ	Jonquière, Que., Canada
JGA	Jamnagar, India	JLN	Joplin, Mo., USA
YJA	Jasper, Alta., Canada	JUJ	Jujuy, Provincia Jujuy, Argentina (El Cadillal)
JED	Jeddah, Saudi Arabia	JUL	Juliaca, Peru
XRY	Jerez de la Frontera, Spain	JNU	Juneau, Alaska, USA
JER	Jersey, Channel Islands (States)	KOJ	Kagoshima, Japan
JDH	Jodhpur, India	OGG	Kahului, Hawaii, USA

Code	Airport	Code	Airport
KAT	Kaitaia, New Zealand	KAB	Kariba, Zimbabwe
KAE	Kake, Alaska, USA	AOK	Karpathos, Greece
AZO	Kalamazoo, Mich., USA (Kalamazoo/ Battle Creek)	KRP	Karup, Denmark
		BBK	Kasane, Botswana
KLO	Kalibo, Philippines	KSJ	Kasos Island, Greece
KGD	Kaliningrad, Russia	KTR	Katherine, N.T., Australia (Tindal)
FCA	Kalispell, Mont., USA (Glacier Park)	KTM	Kathmandu, Nepal (Tribhuvan)
KLR	Kalmar, Sweden	KTW	Katowice, Poland (Pyrzowice)
KAL	Kaltag, Alaska, USA	LIH	Kauai Island, Hawaii, USA (Lihue Municipal)
YKA	Kamloops, B.C., Canada		
SFJ	Kangerlussuaq, Greenland (Sondre Stromfjord)	HPV	Kauai Island, Hawaii, USA (Princeville)
KAN	Kano, Nigeria (Aminu Kano)	KUN	Kaunas, Lithuania
MKC	Kansas City, Mo., USA (Downtown)	KVA	Kavala, Greece
MCI	Kansas City, Mo., USA (International)	KZN	Kazan, Russia
		EAR	Kearney, Nebr., USA
KHH	Kaohsiung, Taiwan	EEN	Keene/Brattleboro, N.H., USA (Dillant Hopkins)
JHM	Kapalua, Hawaii, USA		
YYU	Kapuskasing, Ont., Canada	YLW	Kelowna, B.C., Canada (Ellison Field)
KHI	Karachi, Pakistan	KEJ	Kemerovo, Russia

Code	Airport
KEM	Kemi/Tornio, Finland
ENA	Kenai, Alaska, USA
KEH	Kenmore Air Harbor, Wash., USA
YQK	Kenora, Ont., Canada
CFU	Kerkyra, Greece
KER	Kerman, Iran
KSH	Kermanshah, Iran (Bakhtaran Iran)
KTN	Ketchikan, Alaska, USA
EYW	Key West, Fla., USA
KHV	Khabarovsk, Russia (Novy)
HRK	Kharkov, Ukraine
KRT	Khartoum, Sudan
KEL	Kiel, Germany (Holtenau)
KBP	Kiev, Ukraine (Borispol)
IEV	Kiev, Ukraine (Zhulhany)
TKQ	Kigoma, Tanzania
JRO	Kilimanjaro, Tanzania
ILE	Killeen, Tex., USA
KNS	King Island, Tas., Australia

Code	Airport
IGM	Kingman, Ariz., USA (Mohave County)
KGC	Kingscote, S.A., Australia
KIN	Kingston, Jamaica
YGK	Kingston, Ont., Canada
FIH	Kinshasa, Zaire
ISO	Kinston, N.C., USA
KPN	Kipnuk, Alaska, USA
KKN	Kirkenes, Norway (Høeyburtmøen)
KOI	Kirkwall, Orkney Island, Scotland
KRN	Kiruna, Sweden
KIV	Kishinev, Moldova
YKF	Kitchener, Ont., Canada
KLU	Klagenfurt, Austria
LMT	Klamath Falls, Oreg., USA (Kingsley Field)
KLW	Klawock, Alaska, USA
TYS	Knoxville, Tenn., USA (McGhee Tyson)
ADQ	Kodiak, Alaska, USA

Code	Airport
USM	Koh Samui, Thailand
KOK	Kokkola/Pietarsaari, Finland (Kruunupyy)
KOA	Kona, Hawaii, USA (Keahole)
ROR	Koror, Palau (Airai)
KSC	Košice, Slovakia (Barca)
KSA	Kosrae, Caroline Islands, Micronesia
KBR	Kota Baharu, Malaysia (Sultan Ismail Petra)
BKI	Kota Kinabalu, Sabah, Malaysia
OTZ	Kotzebue, Alaska, USA
KRK	Kraków, Poland (Balice)
KRF	Kramfors, Sweden
KRR	Krasnodar, Russia
KJA	Krasnojarsk, Russia
KRS	Kristiansand, Norway (Kjevik)
KSU	Kristiansund, Norway (Kvernberget)
KUL	Kuala Lumpur, Malaysia
TGG	Kuala Terengganu, Malaysia (Sultan Mahmood)

Code	Airport
KUA	Kuantan, Malaysia (Padang Geroda)
KCH	Kuching, Sarawak, Malaysia
KUS	Kulusuk, Greenland
KMJ	Kumamoto, Japan
KMG	Kunming, China
KUV	Kunsan, South Korea
KUO	Kuopio, Finland
YVP	Kuujjuaq, Que., Canada (Fort Chimo)
YGW	Kuujjuarapik, Que., Canada
KWI	Kuwait, Kuwait
KWA	Kwajalein, Marshall Islands
LCE	La Ceiba, Honduras
LCG	La Coruña, Spain
LSE	La Crosse, Wis., USA
LAP	La Paz, Baja California Sur, Mexico
LPB	La Paz, Bolivia (El Alto)
LRH	La Rochelle, France (Laleu)
YVC	La Ronge, Sask., Canada
SSQ	La Sarre, Que., Canada

Code	Airport
LSC	La Serena, Chile (La Florida)
YLQ	La Tuque, Que., Canada
EUN	Laayoune, Morocco
LBU	Labuan, Sabah, Malaysia
XEE	Lac Édouard, Que., Canada
XEH	Ladysmith, B.C., Canada
LAF	Lafayette, Ind., USA (Purdue University)
LFT	Lafayette/New Iberia, La., USA
LOS	Lagos, Nigeria (Murtala Muhammed)
LDU	Lahad Datu, Sabah, Malaysia
LHE	Lahore, Pakistan
LCH	Lake Charles, La., USA
LKL	Lakselv, Norway
LNY	Lanai City, Hawaii, USA
LNS	Lancaster, Pa., USA
XEJ	Langford, B.C., Canada
LGK	Langkawi, Malaysia
LAN	Lansing, Mich., USA (Capital City)

Code	Airport
ACE	Lanzarote, Canary Islands, Spain
LAR	Laramie, Wyo., USA (General Brees Field)
LRD	Laredo, Tex., USA
LCA	Larnaca, Cyprus
LRU	Las Cruces, N. Mex., USA
LSP	Las Piedras, Venezuela (Josefa Camejo)
LAS	Las Vegas, Nev., USA (McCarran International)
VGT	Las Vegas, Nev., USA (North Air Terminal)
LBE	Latrobe, Pa., USA (Westmoreland County)
LST	Launceston, Tas., Australia
PIB	Laurel, Miss., USA (L'l Hattiesburg/ Camp Shelby)
LWY	Lawas, Sarawak, Malaysia
LAW	Lawton, Okla., USA
LZC	Lazaro Cardenas, Michoacan, Mexico
LEH	Le Havre, France

Code	Airport	Code	Airport
LEA	Learmonth, W.A., Australia	LGG	Liège, Belgium (Bierset)
LEB	Lebanon/Hanover/White River, N.H., USA	LLW	Lilongwe, Malawi (Kamuzu)
		LIM	Lima, Peru (International Jorge Chávez)
LBA	Leeds/Bradford, England		
LGP	Legaspi, Philippines	LMN	Limbang, Sarawak, Malaysia
LEJ	Leipzig, Germany	LIG	Limoges, France (Bellegarde)
LKN	Leknes, Norway	LNK	Lincoln, Nebr., USA
BJX	León/Guanajuato, Guanajuato, Mexico (Del Bajio)	LPI	Linköping, Sweden (Saab)
		LNZ	Linz, Austria
LRS	Leros, Greece	LIS	Lisbon, Portugal
YQL	Lethbridge, Alta., Canada	LSY	Lismore, N.S.W., Australia
LET	Leticia, Colombia (Gen. Av Cob)	LIT	Little Rock, Ark., USA
LWS	Lewiston, Ind., USA (Lewiston–Nez Perce)	LPL	Liverpool, England
		LVI	Livingstone, Zambia
LWT	Lewistown, Mont., USA	LJU	Ljubljana, Slovenia (Brnik)
LEX	Lexington, Ky., USA (Blue Grass Field)	LFW	Lomé, Togo
LBL	Liberal, Kans., USA (Glenn L. Martin)	LNV	Londolovit, Papua New Guinea
LIR	Liberia, Costa Rica	LCY	London, England (City)
LBV	Libreville, Gabon	LGW	London, England (Gatwick)

Code	Airport	Code	Airport
LHR	London, England (Heathrow)	LUD	Luderitz, Namibia
LTN	London, England (Luton)	LUG	Lugano, Switzerland (Agno)
STN	London, England (Stansted)	VSG	Lugansk, Ukraine
YXU	London, Ont., Canada	LUA	Lukla, Nepal
LDB	Londrina, Paraná, Brazil	LLA	Lulea, Sweden (Kallax)
LGB	Long Beach, Calif., USA	LUN	Lusaka, Zambia
GGG	Longview/Gladewater/Kilgore, Tex., USA	LUX	Luxembourg, Luxembourg (Findel)
		LXR	Luxor, Egypt
LYR	Longyearbyen, Norway (Svalbard)	LWO	Lvov, Ukraine (Snilow)
LTO	Loreto, Baja California Sur, Mexico	LYH	Lynchburg, Va., USA
LRT	Lorient, France (Lann-Bihoue)	LYS	Lyon, France (Satolas)
LAX	Los Angeles, Calif., USA	MST	Maastricht, Netherlands (Zuid-Limburg)
LSQ	Los Angeles, Chile (María Dolores)		
LMM	Los Mochis, Sinaloa, Mexico	MFE	McAllen/Mission, Tex., USA
SDF	Louisville, Ky., USA (Standiford Field)	MCK	McCook, Nebr., USA
LDE	Lourdes/Tarbes, France	MCG	McGrath, Alaska, USA
LAD	Luanda, Angola (Fevereiro)	MCP	Macapá, Amapá, Brazil
LBB	Lubbock, Tex., USA	MKY	Mackay, Queensland, Australia
LKO	Lucknow, India	MCN	Macon, Ga., USA (Lewis B. Wilson)

Code	Airport
MAG	Madang, Papua New Guinea
MSN	Madison, Wis., USA (Dane County)
MAA	Madras, India (Meenambarkkam)
MAD	Madrid, Spain (Barajas)
IXM	Madurai, India
HGN	Mae Hong Son, Thailand
GDX	Magadan, Russia
SEZ	Mahe Island, Seychelles
MAJ	Majuro, Marshall Islands
SSG	Malabo, Equatorial Guinea (Santa Isabel)
AGP	Málaga, Spain
MLG	Malang, Indonesia
MLE	Malé, Maldives
HMA	Malmö, Sweden (Malmö Harbour)
JMM	Malmö, Sweden (Malmö Harbour Heliport)
MMX	Malmö, Sweden (Sturup)
PTF	Malololailai, Fiji

Code	Airport
MLA	Malta, Malta (Luqa)
MMH	Mammoth Lakes, Calif., USA
MDC	Manado, Indonesia (Samratulang)
MGA	Managua, Nicaragua
MAO	Manaus, Amazonas, Brazil (Eduardo Gomes)
MAN	Manchester, England (Ringway)
MHT	Manchester, N.H., USA
IXE	Mangalore, India (Bajpe)
MAY	Mangrove Cay, Bahamas
MHK	Manhattan, Kans., USA
MNL	Manila, Philippines (Ninoy Aquino)
MBL	Manistee, Mich., USA
MZL	Manizales, Colombia (Santaguida)
MKW	Manokwari, Indonesia (Rendani)
ZLO	Manzanillo, Colima, Mexico
MPM	Maputo, Mozambique
MDQ	Mar del Plata, Buenos Aires, Argentina

Code	Airport
MAR	Maracaibo, Venezuela (La Chinita)
MTH	Marathon, Fla., USA
YSP	Marathon, Ont., Canada
MRK	Marco Island, Fla., USA
MHQ	Mariehamn, Åland Island, Finland
MWA	Marion, Ill., USA
MQT	Marquette, Mich., USA
RAK	Marrakech, Morocco (Menara)
MRS	Marseille, France
MHH	Marsh Harbour, Bahamas
MVY	Martha's Vineyard, Mass., USA
MSU	Maseru, Lesotho
MCW	Mason City, Iowa, USA
MSS	Massena, N.Y., USA
MAM	Matamoros, Tamaulipas, Mexico
AMI	Mataram, Indonesia (Selaparang)
MYJ	Matsuyama, Japan
MUN	Maturin, Venezuela
MUB	Maun, Botswana

Code	Airport
MRU	Mauritius, Mauritius (Plaisance)
XID	Maxville, Ont., Canada
MAZ	Mayaguez, P.R., USA (El Maui)
MZT	Mazatlán, Sinaloa, Mexico (Buelna)
MES	Medan, Indonesia (Polonia)
EOH	Medellín, Colombia (Enrique Olaya Herrara)
MDE	Medellín, Colombia (La Playas)
MFR	Medford, Oreg., USA (Medford/Jackson County)
YXH	Medicine Hat, Alta., Canada
MED	Medina, Saudi Arabia
MEY	Meghauli, Nepal
MLB	Melbourne, Fla., USA
MEL	Melbourne, Vic., Australia (Tullamarine)
XEK	Melville, Sask., Canada
MMB	Memanbetsu, Japan
MEM	Memphis, Tenn., USA
MDZ	Mendoza, Argentina (El Plumerillo)

Code	Airport
MNM	Menominee, Mich., USA
MAH	Menorca, Spain
MRD	Mérida, Venezuela (Alberto Carnevalli)
MID	Merida, Yucatan, Mexico
MEI	Meridian, Miss., USA (Key Field)
ETZ	Metz/Nancy, France (Frescaty)
MXL	Mexicali, Baja California, Mexico
MEX	Mexico City, Distrito Federal, Mexico
MIA	Miami, Fla., USA (International)
OPF	Miami, Fla., USA (Opa Locka)
MPB	Miami, Fla., USA (Public Seaplane Base)
MBS	Midland/Bay City/Saginaw, Mich., USA
MAF	Midland/Odessa, Tex., USA
JMK	Mikonos, Greece
LIN	Milan, Italy (Linate)
MXP	Milan, Italy (Malpensa)
BGY	Milan, Italy (Orio al Serio)

Code	Airport
MQL	Mildura, Vic., Australia
MLS	Miles City, Mont., USA
MFN	Milford Sound, New Zealand
MLO	Milos, Greece
MKE	Milwaukee, Wis., USA (General Mitchell Field)
MSP	Minneapolis, Minn., USA (Minneapolis/St Paul)
MOT	Minot, N.Dak., USA
MSQ	Minsk, Belarus
MYY	Miri, Sarawak, Malaysia
MSJ	Misawa, Japan
MSO	Missoula, Mont., USA
KMI	Miyazaki, Japan
MQN	Mo I Rana, Norway (Rossvoll)
CNY	Moab, Utah, USA
MOB	Mobile, Ala., USA
MOD	Modesto, Calif., USA (Harry Sham Field)
MGQ	Mogadishu, Somalia

Code	Airport
NWA	Moheli, Comoros
MOL	Molde, Norway (Arø)
MLI	Moline, Ill., USA (Quad City)
MBA	Mombasa, Kenya (Moi International)
MIR	Monastir, Tunisia (Skanes)
LOV	Monclova, Coahuila, Mexico
YQM	Moncton, N.B., Canada (Lakeburn)
MLU	Monroe, La., USA
YYY	Mont Joli, Que., Canada
MCM	Monte Carlo, Monaco
MBJ	Montego Bay, Jamaica (Sangster)
MRY	Monterey/Carmel, Calif., USA
MTY	Monterrey, Nuevo León, Mexico (Escobedo)
MVD	Montevideo, Uruguay (Carrasco)
MGM	Montgomery, Ala., USA (Dannelly Field)
MPL	Montpellier, France (Fréjorgues)
YUL	Montreal, Dorval, Canada

Code	Airport
YMX	Montreal, Mirabel, Canada
MTJ	Montrose, Colo., USA
MNI	Montserrat, Montserrat (Blackburne)
YMO	Moosonee, Ont., Canada
MLM	Morelia, Michoacan, Mexico
MGW	Morgantown, W.Va., USA
HNA	Morioka, Japan (Hanamaki)
ONG	Mornington, Qld., Australia
HAH	Moroni, Comoros (Hahaya)
YVA	Moroni, Comoros (Hahaya/Iconi)
MMU	Morristown, N.J., USA
MYA	Moruya, N.S.W., Australia
MOW	Moscow, Russia
DME	Moscow, Russia (Domodedovo)
SVO	Moscow, Russia (Sheremetyevo)
VKO	Moscow, Russia (Vnukovo)
LLY	Mount Holly, N.J., USA
MVN	Mount Vernon, Ill., USA
WMH	Mountain Home, Ark., USA

Code	Airport
MPA	Mpacha, Namibia
MKM	Mukah, Sarawak, Malaysia
MLH	Mulhouse, France
MZV	Mulu, Malaysia
MIE	Muncie, Ind., USA (Delaware County)
MUC	Munich, Germany (Franz Josef Strauss)
FMO	Münster, Germany
MJV	Murcia, Spain (San Javier)
MMK	Murmansk, Russia
MCT	Muscat, Oman (Seeb)
MSL	Muscle Shoals/Florence/Sheffield, Ala., USA
MKG	Muskegon, Mich., USA
MYR	Myrtle Beach, S.C., USA
MJT	Mytilene, Greece
NAN	Nadi, Fiji
NGS	Nagasaki, Japan
NGO	Nagoya, Japan (Komaki)

Code	Airport
NAG	Nagpur, India (Sonegaon)
NAH	Naha, Indonesia
NBO	Nairobi, Kenya (Jomo Kenyatta)
WIL	Nairobi, Kenya (Wilson)
NAK	Nakhon Ratchasima, Thailand
APL	Nampula, Mozambique
ZNA	Nanaimo, B.C., Canada
YCD	Nanaimo, B.C., Canada (Cassidy)
NKG	Nanjing, China
NNG	Nanning, China
NTE	Nantes, France (Nantes-Château Bougon)
ACK	Nantucket, Mass., USA
WNA	Napakiak, Alaska, USA
APF	Naples, Fla., USA
NAP	Naples, Italy (Capodichino)
UAK	Narsarsuaq, Greenland
JNS	Narssaq, Greenland
BNA	Nashville, Tenn., USA

Code	Airport	Code	Airport
NAS	Nassau, Bahamas (International)	MSY	New Orleans, La., USA (Moisant)
PID	Nassau, Bahamas (Paradise Island)	NPL	New Plymouth, New Zealand
NAT	Natal, Rio Grande do Norte, Brazil	XEM	New Richmond, Que., Canada
INU	Nauru, Nauru	TSS	New York, N.Y., USA (E. 34th Street Heliport)
NVT	Navegantes, Santa Catarina, Brazil		
JNX	Naxos, Cyclades Islands, Greece	JFK	New York, N.Y., USA (John F. Kennedy)
NDJ	N'Djamena, Chad	LGA	New York, N.Y., USA (La Guardia)
NLA	Ndola, Zambia	JRA	New York, N.Y., USA (City)
NEC	Necochea, Buenos Aires, Argentina	EWR	Newark, N.J., USA
NSN	Nelson, New Zealand	SWF	Newburgh/Poughkeepsie, N.Y., USA (Stewart)
NLP	Nelspruit, South Africa		
KEP	Nepalganj, Nepal	NCL	Newcastle, England
NEV	Nevis, Leeward Islands, Saint Kitts and Nevis	XEY	Newcastle, N.B., Canada
		BEO	Newcastle, N.S.W., Australia (Belmont)
EWB	New Bedford/Fall River, Mass., USA	NTL	Newcastle, N.S.W., Australia (Williamtown)
EWN	New Bern, N.C., USA (Simmons–Nott)		
		ZNE	Newman, W.A., Australia
XEL	New Carlisle, Que., Canada	PHF	Newport News/Williamsburg/Hampton Va., USA
HVN	New Haven, Conn., USA		

Code	Airport	Code	Airport
NQY	Newquay, England	OVB	Novosibirsk, Russia (Tolmachevo)
XLV	Niagara Falls, Ont., Canada	NLD	Nuevo Laredo, Tamaulipas, Mexico
NCE	Nice, France (Côte d'Azur)	TBU	Nuku Alofa/Tongatapu, Tonga
NJC	Nizhnevartovsk, Russia	NUE	Nuremberg, Germany
GOJ	Nizhniy Novgorod, Russia	GOH	Nuuk, Greenland
OME	Nome, Alaska, USA	ODW	Oak Harbor, Wash., USA
OFK	Norfolk, Nebr., USA (Karl Stefan)	OAK	Oakland, Calif., USA
ORF	Norfolk, Va., USA	XOK	Oakville, Ont., Canada
YYB	North Bay, Ont., Canada (Jack Garland)	OAX	Oaxaca, Oaxaca, Mexico (Xoxocotlan)
OTH	North Bend, Oreg., USA	OBO	Obihiro, Japan
NCA	North Caicos, Turks and Caicos Islands	ODE	Odense, Denmark
ELH	North Eleuthera, Bahamas	ODS	Odessa, Ukraine
LBF	North Platte, Nebr., USA (Lee Bird Field)	OGS	Ogdensburg, N.Y., USA
		OHD	Ohrid, Macedonia
NWI	Norwich, England	OIT	Oita, Japan
OWD	Norwood, Mass., USA	OKJ	Okayama, Japan
NKC	Nouakchott, Mauritania	OKA	Okinawa, Ryukyu Islands, Japan (Naha Field)
NOU	Noumea, New Caledonia (Tontouta)		

Code	Airport
OKC	Oklahoma City, Okla., USA (Will Rogers)
OMA	Omaha, Nebr., USA (Eppley Airfield)
ONT	Ontario, Calif., USA
OPO	Oporto, Portugal
OMR	Oradea, Romania
ORN	Oran, Algeria (Es Senia)
OAG	Orange, N.S.W., Australia (Springhill)
ORB	Örebro, Sweden
ORL	Orlando, Fla., USA (Herndon)
MCO	Orlando, Fla., USA (International)
ITM	Osaka, Japan (Itami International)
KIX	Osaka, Japan (Kansai International)
OSA	Osaka, Japan (Osaka International)
YOO	Oshawa, Ont., Canada
OSH	Oshkosh, Wis., USA (Wittman Field)
FBU	Oslo, Norway (Fornebu)
GEN	Oslo, Norway (Garderm)
OSD	Östersund, Sweden (Froesoe)

Code	Airport
YOW	Ottawa, Ont., Canada
OTM	Ottumwa, Iowa, USA
OUA	Ouagadougou, Burkina Faso
OZZ	Ouarzazate, Morocco
OUL	Oulu, Finland
VDA	Ovda, Israel
OWB	Owensboro, Ky., USA
OXR	Oxnard/Ventura, Calif., USA
PDG	Padang, Indonesia (Tabing)
PAD	Paderborn, Germany
PAH	Paducah, Ky., USA
PGA	Page, Ariz., USA
PPG	Pago Pago, American Samoa
PLQ	Palanga, Lithuania
PLM	Palembang, Indonesia
PMO	Palermo, Sicily, Italy (Punta Raisi)
PSP	Palm Springs, Calif., USA
PMI	Palma, Mallorca, Spain
PMD	Palmdale, Calif., USA

Code	Airport
PMR	Palmerston North, New Zealand
PLW	Palu, Indonesia (Mutiara)
PNA	Pamplona, Spain
PFN	Panama City, Fla., USA
PTY	Panama City, Panama (Tocumen)
PJG	Panjgur, Pakistan
PNL	Pantelleria, Italy
PPT	Papeete, French Polynesia
PFO	Paphos, Cyprus
PBO	Paraburdoo, W.A., Australia
PBM	Paramaribo, Suriname (Zanderij)
XFE	Parent, Que., Canada
PAR	Paris, France
CDG	Paris, France (Charles De Gaulle)
JDP	Paris, France (Issy-les-Moulineaux)
ORY	Paris, France (Orly)
PKB	Parkersburg/Marietta, W.Va., USA (Wood County)
PKE	Parkes, N.S.W., Australia

Code	Airport
XPB	Parksville, B.C., Canada
PAS	Páros, Greece
PSO	Pasto, Colombia (Cano)
PAT	Patna, India
YPE	Peace River, Alta., Canada
PKU	Pekanbaru, Indonesia (Simpang Tiga)
PLN	Pellston, Mich., USA
YTA	Pembroke, Ontario, Canada
PEN	Penang, Malaysia
PDT	Pendleton Oreg., USA
PNS	Pensacola, Fla., USA
YYF	Penticton, B.C., Canada
PZE	Penzance, England
PIA	Peoria, Ill., USA
XFG	Perce, Que., Canada
PEI	Pereira, Colombia (Matecana)
PGX	Périgueux, France
PEE	Perm, Russia

Code	Airport	Code	Airport
PGF	Perpignan, France (Llabanere)	THU	Pituffik, Greenland (Thule)
PER	Perth, W.A., Australia	PLB	Plattsburgh, N.Y., USA
PEG	Perugia, Italy	PLH	Plymouth, England
PSR	Pescara, Italy (Liberi)	PIH	Pocatello, Idaho, USA
PEW	Peshawar, Pakistan	TGD	Podgorica, Yugoslavia (Golubovci)
PSG	Petersburg, Alaska, USA	KPO	Pohang, South Korea
PKC	Petropavlovsk-Kamchatsky, Russia	PNI	Pohnpei, Caroline Islands, Micronesia
PES	Petrozavodsk, Russia	PHO	Point Hope, Alaska, USA
PHL	Philadelphia, Pa., USA	PTP	Pointe-à-Pitre, Guadeloupe (Le Raizet)
PHS	Phitsanulok, Thailand		
PNH	Phnom Penh, Cambodia (Pochentong)	XPX	Pointe-aux-Trembles, Que., Canada
		PNR	Pointe Noire, Congo
PHX	Phoenix, Ariz., USA (Sky Harbor)	PKR	Pokhara, Nepal
HKT	Phuket, Thailand	PNC	Ponca City, Okla., USA
PIR	Pierre, S.Dak., USA	PSE	Ponce, P.R., USA (Mercedita)
PTG	Pietersburg, South Africa	PDL	Ponta Delgada, Azores, Portugal (Nordela)
PIW	Pikwitonei, Man., Canada		
PSA	Pisa, Italy (Galileo Galilei)	PNK	Pontianak, Indonesia (Supadio)
PIT	Pittsburgh, Pa., USA	PNQ	Poona, India

Code	Airport	Code	Airport
POR	Pori, Finland	PDX	Portland, Oreg., USA
PMV	Porlamar, Venezuela (Gen. Santiago Marino)	POA	Pôrto Alegre, Rio Grande do Sul, Brazil
CLM	Port Angeles, Wash., USA (William Fairchild)	PXO	Porto Santo, Madeira, Portugal
		PSM	Portsmouth, N.H., USA (Pease)
PAP	Port-au-Prince, Haiti (Mais Gate)	POU	Poughkeepsie, N.Y., USA (Dutchess County)
IXZ	Port Blair, India		
PLZ	Port Elizabeth, South Africa (H. F. Verwoerd)	YPW	Powell River, B.C., Canada
		PAZ	Poza Rica, Veracruz, Mexico
POG	Port Gentil, Gabon	POZ	Poznań, Poland (Lawica)
YZT	Port Hardy, B.C., Canada	PRG	Prague, Czech Republic (Ruzyne)
PHE	Port Hedland, W.A., Australia	PRI	Praslin Island, Seychelles
PLO	Port Lincoln, S.A., Australia	PRC	Prescott, Ariz., USA
PQQ	Port Macquarie, N.S.W., Australia	PQI	Presque Isle, Maine, USA
POM	Port Moresby, Papua New Guinea (Jackson)	YXS	Prince George, B.C., Canada
		YPR	Prince Rupert, B.C., Canada
POS	Port of Spain, Trinidad, Trinidad and Tobago	PCT	Princeton, N.J., USA
		PVD	Providence, R.I., USA (Green State)
VLI	Port Vila, Vanuatu (Bauerfield)	PLS	Providenciales, Turks and Caicos Islands
PWM	Portland, Maine, USA		

Code	Airport
PVC	Provincetown, Mass., USA
PVU	Provo, Utah, USA
PCL	Pucallpa, Peru (Captain Rolden)
PBC	Puebla, Puebla, Mexico
PUB	Pueblo, Colo., USA
PUZ	Puerto Cabezas, Nicaragua
PXM	Puerto Escondido, Oaxaca, Mexico
PMC	Puerto Montt, Chile (Tepual)
PZO	Puerto Ordaz, Venezuela
POP	Puerto Plata, Dominican Republic (La Union)
PPS	Puerto Princesa, Philippines
PSZ	Puerto Suárez, Bolivia
PVR	Puerto Vallarta, Jalisco, Mexico
PUY	Pula, Croatia (Hrvatska)
PUW	Pullman, Wash., USA
PUQ	Punta Arenas, Chile (Presidente Ibanez)
PUJ	Punta Cana, Dominican Republic

Code	Airport
PUS	Pusan, South Korea (Kimhae)
XQU	Qualicum, B.C., Canada
YQC	Quaqtaq, Que., Canada
YQB	Quebec, Que., Canada (Ste-Foy Airport)
ZQN	Queenstown, New Zealand (Frankton)
UEL	Quelimane, Mozambique
XQP	Quepos, Costa Rica
QRO	Queretaro, Queretaro, Mexico
YQZ	Quesnel, B.C., Canada
UET	Quetta, Pakistan
UIB	Quibdo, Colombia
UIP	Quimper, France (Pluguffan)
UIN	Quincy, Ill., USA (Baldwin Field)
UIO	Quito, Ecuador (Mariscal)
RBA	Rabat, Morocco (Sale)
RAB	Rabaul, Papua New Guinea (Lakunai)
YOP	Rainbow Lake, Alta., Canada

Code	Airport
RPR	Raipur, India
RAJ	Rajkot, India
RDU	Raleigh/Durham, N.C., USA
RAP	Rapid City, S.Dak., USA
RAR	Rarotonga, Cook Islands
RDG	Reading, Pa., USA (Municipal/Spaatz Field)
REC	Recife, Pernambuco, Brazil (Guararapes)
YRL	Red Lake, Ont., Canada
RDD	Redding, Calif., USA
REG	Reggio Calabria, Italy (Tito Menniti)
YQR	Regina, Sask., Canada
RNS	Rennes, France (St-Jacques)
RNO	Reno, Nev., USA
RES	Resistencia, Chaco, Argentina
YRB	Resolute, N.W.T., Canada
REU	Reus, Spain
RKV	Reykjavik, Iceland (Domestic)

Code	Airport
KEF	Reykjavik, Iceland (Keflavik)
REX	Reynosa, Tamaulipas, Mexico (Gen. Lucio Blanco)
RHI	Rhinelander, Wis., USA
RHO	Rhodes, Greece (Paradisi)
RCB	Richards Bay, South Africa
RIC	Richmond, Va, USA
RIX	Riga, Latvia
RIO	Rio de Janeiro, Brazil
GIG	Rio de Janeiro, Brazil (International)
SDU	Rio de Janeiro, Brazil (Santos Dumont)
RGL	Rio Gallegos, Santa Cruz, Argentina
RGA	Rio Grande, Tierra Del Fuego, Argentina
RIW	Riverton, Wyo, USA
XRP	Riviere-à-Pierre, Que., Canada
RUH	Riyadh, Saudi Arabia (King Khaled)
ROA	Roanoke, Va., USA
RTB	Roatan, Honduras

Code	Airport	Code	Airport
RCE	Roche Harbor, Wash., USA	ROW	Roswell, N. Mex., USA
RST	Rochester, Minn., USA	ROP	Rota, Northern Mariana Islands
ROC	Rochester, N.Y., USA (Monroe County)	RTM	Rotterdam, Netherlands
		URO	Rouen, France (Rouen/Boos)
RSD	Rock Sound, Bahamas	RUI	Ruidoso, N.Mex., USA
RKS	Rock Springs, Wyo., USA		
		RUT	Rutland, Vt., USA
ZRF	Rockford, Ill., USA		
		SCN	Saarbrücken, Germany (Ensheim)
RFD	Rockford, Ill., USA (Greater Rockford)	SAB	Saba Island, Netherlands Antilles
RKD	Rockland, Maine, USA (Rockland)	SMF	Sacramento, Calif., USA
RWI	Rocky Mount, N.C., USA (Wilson)	SPD	Saidpur, Bangladesh
RRG	Rodrigues Island, Mauritius	SBH	St-Barthélemy, Guadeloupe
RMA	Roma, Qld., Australia	YCM	St Catharine's, Ont., Canada
CIA	Rome, Italy (Ciampino)	STC	St Cloud, Minn., USA
FCO	Rome, Italy (Leonardo da Vinci/ Fiumicino)	STX	St Croix Island, V.I., USA
		SSB	St Croix Island, V.I., USA (Sea Plane Base)
RNB	Ronneby, Sweden (Kallinge)		
ROS	Rosario, Santa Fe, Argentina (Fisherton)	RUN	St-Denis de la Réunion, Réunion (Gillot)
ROV	Rostov, Russia	SGO	St George, Qld., Australia

Code	Airport	Code	Airport
SGU	St George, Utah, USA	LED	St Petersburg, Russia (Pulkovo)
GND	St Georges, Grenada (Pt Saline)	PIE	St Petersburg/Clearwater, Fla., USA
XIM	St-Hyacinthe, Que., Canada	FSP	St-Pierre, St-Pierre and Miquelon
YYT	St John's, Newfoundland, Canada	STT	St Thomas Island, V.I., USA (Cyril E. King)
ANU	St John's/Antigua, Antigua and Barbuda	SPB	St Thomas Island, V.I., USA (Seaplane Base)
YSJ	St John, N.B., Canada	SVD	St Vincent, St Vincent and the Grenadines
SKB	St Kitts, Saint Kitts and Nevis (Golden Rock)	SPN	Saipan, Northern Mariana Islands
YSL	St Leonard, N.B., Canada	SNO	Sakon Nakhon, Thailand
STL	St Louis, Mo., USA (Lambert–St Louis)	SID	Sal, Cape Verde (Amilcar Cabral)
UVF	St Lucia, St Lucia (Hewanorra)	SLN	Salina, Kans., USA
SLU	St Lucia, St Lucia (Vigie Field)	SBY	Salisbury, Md., USA
SXM	St Maarten, Netherlands Antilles (Juliana)	YSN	Salmon Arm, B.C., Canada
SFG	St-Martin, Netherlands Antilles (Espérance)	SLC	Salt Lake City, Utah., USA
		SLA	Salta, Argentina
XIO	St Marys, Ont., Canada	SLW	Saltillo, Coahuila, Mexico
STP	St Paul, Minn., USA (Downtown)	SSA	Salvador, Bahía, Brazil (Dois de Julho)

Code	Airport	Code	Airport
SZG	Salzburg, Austria	SJU	San Juan, P.R., USA (Luis Munoz Marin)
KUF	Samara, Russia		
SKD	Samarkand, Uzbekistan	SBP	San Luis Obispo, Calif., USA
ADZ	San Andrés Island, Colombia	SLP	San Luis Potosí, Mexico
SJT	San Angelo, Tex., USA	CPC	San Martín de los Andes, Neuquen, Argentina
SAT	San Antonio, Tex., USA (International)	SPR	San Pedro, Belize
SVZ	San Antonio, Venezuela	SAP	San Pedro Sula, Honduras (La Mesa)
BRC	San Carlos de Bariloche, Rio Negro, Argentina	ZSA	San Salvador, Bahamas
		SAL	San Salvador, El Salvador
SAN	San Diego, Calif., USA (Lindbergh)	EAS	San Sebastián, Spain (Fuenterrabia)
SFO	San Francisco, Calif., USA	SOM	San Tomé, Venezuela
SJO	San José, Costa Rica (Juan Santamaría)	SAH	Sanaa, Yemen
		SDK	Sandakan, Sabah, Malaysia
SJD	San José del Cabo, Baja California Sur, Mexico	SDN	Sandane, Norway
SJC	San Jose, Calif., USA	TRF	Sandefjord, Norway (Torf)
SJI	San Jose, Philippines (McGuire Field)	SSJ	Sandnessjoen, Norway (Stokka)
		SNA	Santa Ana, Calif., USA (John Wayne)
UAQ	San Juan, Argentina	SBA	Santa Barbara, Calif., USA

Code	Airport	Code	Airport
VVI	Santa Cruz, Bolivia (Viru Viru)	SYX	Sanya, China
SPC	Santa Cruz de la Palma, Canary Islands, Spain	SLZ	São Luís, Maranhão, Brazil (Tirirical)
SFN	Santa Fe, Argentina	CGH	São Paulo, São Paulo, Brazil (Congonhas)
SAF	Santa Fe, N. Mex., USA	GRU	São Paulo, São Paulo, Brazil (Guarulhos)
SMX	Santa Maria, Calif., USA		
STS	Santa Rosa, Calif., USA (Sonoma County)	CTS	Sapporo, Japan (Chitose)
RSA	Santa Rosa, La Pampa, Argentina	SJJ	Sarajevo, Bosnia/Hercegovina (Butmir)
SDR	Santander, Spain	SLK	Saranac Lake, N.Y., USA (Adirondack)
STM	Santarem, Pará, Brazil	SRQ	Sarasota/Bradenton, Fla., USA
SCL	Santiago, Chile (Comodoro Arturo Merino Benitez)	YXE	Saskatoon, Sask., Canada
SCU	Santiago, Cuba (Santiago-Antonio Maceo)	CIU	Sault Ste Marie, Mich., USA (Chippewa County)
STI	Santiago, Dominican Republic	YAM	Sault Ste Marie, Ont., Canada
SCQ	Santiago de Compostela, Spain	JMC	Sausalito, Calif., USA (Marin County)
SDQ	Santo Domingo, Dominican Republic	SAV	Savannah, Ga., USA (Travis Field)
STD	Santo Domingo, Venezuela	SVL	Savonlinna, Finland
JTR	Santorini/Thira Island, Greece	SVU	Savusavu, Fiji

Code	Airport
YKL	Schefferville, Que., Canada
BFF	Scottsbluff, Nebr., USA (William B. Heiling)
LKE	Seattle, Wash., USA (Lake Union Sea Plane)
SEA	Seattle, Wash., USA (Seattle Tacoma)
SDX	Sedona, Ariz., USA
SMM	Semporna, Sabah, Malaysia
SDJ	Sendai, Japan
SEL	Seoul, South Korea (Kimpo)
YZV	Sept-Îles, Que., Canada
SVQ	Seville, Spain
SFA	Sfax, Tunisia
SHA	Shanghai, China (Shanghai/ Hongqiao)
SNN	Shannon, Ireland
SWA	Shantou, China
SHJ	Sharjah, United Arab Emirates
SSH	Sharm el Sheikh, Egypt (Ophira)

Code	Airport
XFL	Shawinigan, Que., Canada
XFM	Shawnigan, B.C., Canada
SHE	Shenyang, China
SZX	Shenzhen, China
SHR	Sheridan, Wyo., USA
LSI	Shetland Islands, Scotland
LWK	Shetland Islands, Scotland (Tingwall)
SJW	Shijiazhuang, China
SYZ	Shiraz, Iran
SYO	Shonai, Japan
SOW	Show Low, Ariz., USA
SHV	Shreveport, La., USA
SBW	Sibu, Sarawak, Malaysia
SDY	Sidney, Mont., USA
SIP	Simferopol, Ukraine
SIN	Singapore, Singapore (Changi)
FSD	Sioux Falls, S.Dak., USA (Joe Foss Field)
YXL	Sioux Lookout, Ont., Canada

Code	Airport	Code	Airport
SIT	Sitka, Alaska, USA	TVL	South Lake Tahoe, Calif., USA
VAS	Sivas, Turkey	SOU	Southampton, England (Eastleigh)
SGY	Skagway, Alaska, USA	SOP	Southern Pines, N.C., USA (Pinehurst)
SFT	Skelleftea, Sweden		
JSI	Skiathos, Greece	SPW	Spencer, Iowa, USA
SKP	Skopje, Macedonia	SPU	Split, Croatia (Hrvatska)
SXL	Sligo, Ireland (Collooney)	GEG	Spokane, Wash., USA
YSH	Smith Falls, Ont., Canada	SPI	Springfield, Ill., USA
YYD	Smithers, B.C., Canada	SGF	Springfield, Mo., USA
SNB	Snake Bay, N.T., Australia	SXR	Srinagar, India
SOF	Sofia, Bulgaria	SMS	Ste Marie, Madagascar
SOG	Sogndal, Norway (Haukasen)	SCE	State College, Pa., USA (University Park)
SHO	Sokcho, South Korea	SHD	Staunton, Va., USA (Shenandoah Valley)
SGD	Sønderborg, Denmark		
TZN	South Andros, Bahamas (Congo Town)	SVG	Stavanger, Norway (Sola)
		SML	Stella Maris, Bahamas
SBN	South Bend, Ind., USA (Michiana Regional)	YJT	Stephenville, Nfld., Canada
XSC	South Caicos, Turks and Caicos Islands	ARN	Stockholm, Sweden (Arlanda)
		BMA	Stockholm, Sweden (Bromma)

Code	Airport	Code	Airport
YSF	Stony Rapids, Sask., Canada	YQY	Sydney, N.S., Canada
SYY	Stornoway, Scotland	SYD	Sydney, N.S.W., Australia
SXB	Strasbourg, France (Entzheim)	SYR	Syracuse, N.Y., USA (Hancock)
XFD	Stratford, Ont., Canada	SZZ	Szczecin, Poland (Goleniow)
XTY	Strathroy, Ont., Canada	TBT	Tabatinga, Amazonas, Brazil
SUE	Sturgeon Bay, Wis., USA	TAC	Tacloban, Philippines (Romualdez)
STR	Stuttgart, Germany (Echterdingen)	TAE	Taegu, South Korea
SRE	Sucre, Bolivia	TAG	Tagbilaran, Philippines
YSB	Sudbury, Ont., Canada	TPE	Taipei, Taiwan (Chiang Kai-shek)
SWQ	Sumbawa Island, Indonesia (Brang Bidji)	TSA	Taipei, Taiwan (Sung Shan)
		TYN	Taiyuan, China
SUN	Sun Valley/Hailey, Idaho, USA	TAI	Taiz, Yemen (Al-Janad)
SDL	Sundsvall, Sweden	TLH	Tallahassee, Fla., USA
MCY	Sunshine Coast, Qld., Australia	TLL	Tallinn, Estonia (Ulemiste)
SUB	Surabaya, Indonesia (Juanda)	TPA	Tampa, Fla., USA
URT	Surat Thani, Thailand	TMP	Tampere, Finland (Tampere–Pirkkala)
SGC	Surgut, Russia		
SUV	Suva, Fiji (Nausori)	TAM	Tampico, Tamaulipas, Mexico
SWP	Swakopmund, Namibia	TMW	Tamworth, N.S.W., Australia

Code	Airport
TNG	Tangier, Morocco (Boukhalef Souahel)
TAP	Tapachula, Chiapas, Mexico
TRK	Tarakan, Indonesia
TPP	Tarapoto, Peru
TIZ	Tari, Papua New Guinea
TJA	Tarija, Bolivia
XFO	Taschereau, Que., Canada
TAS	Tashkent, Uzbekistan
TAT	Tatry/Poprad, Slovakia
TUO	Taupo, New Zealand
TRG	Tauranga, New Zealand
TBS	Tbilisi, Georgia (Novo Alexeyevka)
MME	Teesside, England
TGU	Tegucigalpa, Honduras (Toncontin)
THR	Tehran, Iran (Mehrabad)
TLV	Tel Aviv Yafo, Israel (Ben-Gurion)
TEX	Telluride, Colo., USA
TPL	Temple, Tex., USA

Code	Airport
ZCO	Temuco, Chile (Manquehue)
TFN	Tenerife, Canary Islands, Spain (Norte Los Rodeos)
TFS	Tenerife, Canary Islands, Spain (Reina Sofia)
TPQ	Tepic, Nayarit, Mexico
TER	Terceira Island, Azores Islands, Portugal (Lajes)
THE	Teresina, Piaui, Brazil
TTE	Ternate, Indonesia (Babullah)
YXT	Terrace, B.C., Canada
LSS	Terre-de-Haut, Guadeloupe
HUF	Terre Haute, Ind., USA (Hulman Field)
TXK	Texarkana, Ark., USA
TEZ	Tezpur, India (Salonbari)
HAG	The Hague, Netherlands
YQD	The Pas, Man., Canada
SKG	Thessaloníki, Greece
YTD	Thicket Portage, Man., Canada

Code	Airport
TVF	Thief River Falls, Minn., USA
YTH	Thompson, Man., Canada
YQT	Thunder Bay, Ont., Canada
TIS	Thursday Island, Qld., Australia
TIJ	Tijuana, Baja California, Mexico
TSR	Timişoara, Romania
YTS	Timmins, Ont., Canada
TIQ	Tinian, Northern Mariana Islands
TIA	Tirana, Albania (Rinas)
TRE	Tiree, Scotland
TGM	Tîrgu Mureş, Romania
TRZ	Tiruchirapally, India
TIV	Tivat, Yugoslavia
TAB	Tobago, Tobago, Trinidad and Tobago
YAZ	Tofino, B.C., Canada
OOK	Toksook Bay, Alaska, USA
TKS	Tokushima, Japan
NRT	Tokyo, Japan (Narita)

Code	Airport
TOL	Toledo, Ohio, USA
TWB	Toowoomba, Qld., Australia
FOE	Topeka, Kans., USA (Forbes Field)
YTZ	Toronto, Ont., Canada
YYZ	Toronto, Ont., Canada (Pearson International)
TRC	Torreón, Coahuila, Mexico
EIS	Tortola/Beef Island, Virgin Islands
TTJ	Tottori, Japan
TLS	Toulouse, France (Blagnac)
TUF	Tours, France (St-Symphorien)
TSV	Townsville, Qld., Australia
TOY	Toyama, Japan
TZX	Trabzon, Turkey
TPS	Trapani, Sicily, Italy (Birgi)
TVC	Traverse City, Mich., USA (Cherry Capital)
REL	Trelew, Chubut, Argentina
TTN	Trenton, N.J., USA (Mercer County)

Code	Airport	Code	Airport
TRS	Trieste, Italy (Ronchi dei Legionari)	TCL	Tuscaloosa, Ala., USA (Van der Graaff)
TDD	Trinidad, Bolivia		
TRV	Trivandrum, India	TGZ	Tuxtla Gutierrez, Chiapas, Mexico
TOS	Tromsø, Norway (Tromsø/Langes)	TWF	Twin Falls, Idaho, USA
TRD	Trondheim, Norway (Trondheim–Vaernes)	TYR	Tyler, Tex., USA (Pounds Field)
		TJM	Tyumen, Russia
TRU	Trujillo, Peru	UBJ	Ube, Japan
TKK	Truk, Caroline Islands, Micronesia	UDR	Udaipur, India
XLZ	Truro, N.S., Canada	UTH	Udon Thani, Thailand
TUS	Tucson, Ariz., USA	UNT	Uist, Shetland Islands, Scotland
TUC	Tucuman, Argentina (Benjamin Matienzo)	UPG	Ujung Pandang, Indonesia (Hasanudin)
TUL	Tulsa, Okla., USA	ULN	Ulan Bator, Mongolia
TBP	Túmbes, Peru	UUD	Ulan-Ude, Russia
TUN	Tunis, Tunisia (Carthage)	USN	Ulsan, South Korea
TXN	Tunxi, China	ULY	Ulyanovsk, Russia
TUP	Tupelo, Miss., USA (C.D. Lemons)	UME	Umeå, Sweden
TRN	Turin, Italy (Caselle)	UTN	Upington, South Africa
TKU	Turku, Finland	UGC	Urgench, Uzbekistan

Code	Airport
UPN	Uruapan, Michoacan, Mexico
URC	Urumqi, China
USH	Ushuaia, Tierra del Fuego, Argentina
UCA	Utica, N.Y., USA (Oneida County)
VAA	Vaasa, Finland
BDQ	Vadodara, India
VDS	Vadsø, Norway
EGE	Vail/Eagle, Colo., USA
EGE	Vail/Eagle, Colo., USA (Eagle County)
VDZ	Valdez, Alaska, USA
ZAL	Valdivia, Chile (Pichoy)
VLD	Valdosta, Ga., USA
VLC	Valencia, Spain
VLN	Valencia, Venezuela
VLL	Valladolid, Spain
VUP	Valledupar, Colombia
VPS	Valparaiso, Fla., USA (Fort Walton Beach)
CXH	Vancouver, B.C., Canada (Harbour)

Code	Airport
YVR	Vancouver, B.C., Canada (International)
VRA	Varadero, Cuba (Juan Gualberto Gómez)
VNS	Varanasi, India (Babatpur)
VRK	Varkaus, Finland
VAR	Varna, Bulgaria
VST	Västerås, Sweden (Hasslo)
VXO	Växjö, Sweden
VCE	Venice, Italy (Marco Polo)
VER	Veracruz, Veracruz, Mexico
VRB	Vero Beach, Fla., USA
VRN	Verona, Italy
VEY	Vestmannaeyjar, Iceland
VFA	Victoria Falls, Zimbabwe
YYJ	Victoria, B.C., Canada
YWH	Victoria, B.C., Canada (Harbour)
VCT	Victoria, Tex., USA
VIE	Vienna, Austria (Schwechat)

Code	Airport	Code	Airport
VTE	Vientiane, Laos (Wattay)	WGE	Walgett, N.S.W., Australia
VGO	Vigo, Spain	ALW	Walla Walla, Wash., USA
VLG	Villa Gesell, Buenos Aires, Argentina	WAW	Warsaw, Poland (Okecie)
VSA	Villahermosa, Tabasco, Mexico	IAD	Washington, D.C., USA (Dulles)
VNO	Vilnius, Lithuania	DCA	Washington, D.C., USA (National)
VIJ	Virgin Gorda, Virgin Islands	YKQ	Waskaganish, Que., Canada
VIS	Visalia, Calif., USA	WAT	Waterford, Ireland
VBY	Visby, Sweden	ALO	Waterloo, Iowa, USA
VTZ	Vishakhapatnam, India	ART	Watertown, N.Y., USA
VIX	Vitória, Espírito Santo, Brazil	ATY	Watertown, S.Dak., USA
VIT	Vitoria, Spain	YQH	Watson Lake, Y.T., Canada
VVO	Vladivostok, Russia	CWA	Wausau, Wis., USA (Central Wisconsin)
SKS	Vojens Lufthavn, Denmark (Jojens)	YXZ	Wawa, Ont., Canada
VOG	Volgograd, Russia	WLG	Wellington, New Zealand
YWK	Wabush, Nfld., Canada	EAT	Wenatchee Wash., USA (Pangborn Memorial)
ACT	Waco, Tex., USA (Madison Cooper)		
WGA	Wagga-Wagga, N.S.W., Australia	PBI	West Palm Beach, Fla., USA
AIN	Wainwright, Alaska, USA	HPN	Westchester County, N.Y., USA

Code	Airport	Code	Airport
GWT	Westerland, Germany	INT	Winston-Salem, N.C., USA (Smith Reynolds)
XFQ	Weymont, Que., Canada		
YWR	White River, Ont., Canada	WIN	Winton, Qld., Australia
YXY	Whitehorse, Y.T., Canada	OLF	Wolf Point, Mont., USA
SPS	Wichita Falls, Tex., USA	XIP	Woodstock, Ont., Canada
ICT	Wichita, Kans., USA (Mid-Continent)	UMR	Woomera, S.A., Australia
WIC	Wick, Scotland	ORH	Worcester, Mass., USA (James D. O'Brien Field)
AVP	Wilkes Barre/Scranton, Pa., USA		
CUR	Willemstad/Curaçao, Netherlands Antilles	WRL	Worland, Wyo., USA
		WRO	Wrocław, Poland (Strachowice)
YWL	Williams Lake, B.C., Canada	XWY	Wyoming, Ont., Canada
IPT	Williamsport, Pa., USA (Williamsport Lycoming)	XIY	Xi An, China (Xianyang)
		XMN	Xiamen, China
ISN	Williston, N.Dak., USA (Sloulin Field)	YKM	Yakima, Wash., USA
ILM	Wilmington N.C., USA (New Hanover County)	YKS	Yakutsk, Russia
ERS	Windhoek, Namibia (Eros)	GAJ	Yamagata, Japan (Junmachi)
WDH	Windhoek, Namibia (JG Strijdom)	RGN	Yangon, Myanmar (Mingaladon)
YQG	Windsor, Ontario, Canada	NSI	Yaoundé, Cameroon (Nsimalen)
YWG	Winnipeg, Manitoba, Canada	YAP	Yap, Caroline Islands, Micronesia

Code	Airport	Code	Airport
YQI	Yarmouth, Nova Scotia, Canada	ZAG	Zagreb, Croatia (Hrvatska)
YEC	Yechon, South Korea	ZAH	Zahedan, Iran
YZF	Yellowknife, N.W.T., Canada	ZTH	Zákinthos, Greece
EVN	Yerevan, Armenia	ZAM	Zamboanga, Philippines
JOG	Yogyakarta, Indonesia	ZNZ	Zanzibar, Tanzania (Kisauni)
RSU	Yosu, South Korea	ZAZ	Zaragoza, Spain
YNG	Youngstown, Ohio, USA	ZHA	Zhanjiang, China
YUM	Yuma, Ariz., USA	CGO	Zhengzhou, China
ZCL	Zacatecas, Mexico	ZRH	Zurich, Switzerland

Appendix 9 Surviving the Hotel

Once you reach your room, there is a simple safety routine to go through. Make it a ritual, just as airline crew do. Do it straight away when you arrive – don't unpack or do anything else first.

Start by checking the fire notice that is normally on the back of the door. Orient yourself to where the fire escapes are. Enough? No. It's one thing to look at a map, another to see the situation for real. Go out of your door (remembering to lock up) and follow the route to the fire escape. It's so easy to know only the way to the lifts, but you won't be able to use these in an emergency. The UK Fire Brigade has recently been encouraging people to have a plan in place for getting out of their homes in case of fire – this is doubly valuable in a strange location like a hotel.

Imagine that you have to get to the fire escape in the dark through smoke. Count doors along the way. Try to fix any obstacles in your mind. When you reach the fire-escape door, make sure it opens. Horrendously, it has occasionally happened that, when a fire has broken out, guests have been trapped in a hotel because the fire door was kept locked 'for security reasons'. Hold the door open so you don't get stuck, and take a look into the stairwell to get a basic feeling for what the exit route is like.

What if the fire exit is alarmed? Let reception know, then try it anyway. This takes guts to do, but which would you rather be, slightly embarrassed or crisped? A final precaution is to check out your exit in another direction, in case the corridor is blocked.

While you are on your fire-escape patrol, look out for fire aids – hose reels, extinguishers and the like – along the hotel walls.

To help with your hotel safety, carry a small torch (flashlight). If you do have to make that journey to the fire exit at night it is possible that the lights will be out. Many hotels have no natural lighting in the corridors. Unless you have your own torch you are likely to be feeling your way to the exit. Put the torch and the key together by your bedside. Make this another habit – always put them in the same place, so you can find them if you are woken by an alarm in the middle of the night.

Raising the alarm

If a fire alarm sounds, take it seriously. Assume you haven't got long. But bear in mind that you may have to stand outside the building for some time, whatever the weather. Grab some appropriate clothing. If you are the one who spots the fire, or just smells smoke, give reception a call. Don't assume someone else will do it. Take your key. Arrange to meet up with any others in your party at an obvious landmark outside. Then it's time to go. But don't just fling your door open. If there is fire in the corridor outside, the door may be the only thing between you and death. Opening it is inviting the smoke and flames in.

Feel the door to see if it is hot (try both the door surface and the metal furniture like the handle). It's a good idea to use the back of your hand for this – this way, if you don't feel the heat in time and end up getting burned, your palm will still be functional to grab on to things as you go. If the surface is hot, don't open the door. If it is cool, get down low and cautiously open the door, being prepared to slam it if there's trouble. If it seems OK in the corridor, get out and close the door behind you – opportunistic thieves have been known to set off an alarm and then help themselves to the contents of unlocked rooms. And don't try to use the lifts. They should never be used in an emergency evacuation, and you will just waste time heading for them. If you encounter thick smoke, assume the worst and backtrack if necessary.

If smoke or heat results in your being trapped in your room, use wet towels to try to seal vents and cracks where smoke can get in. Phone down to reception or direct to the fire brigade. Signal from your window as dramatically as you can, but don't open the window or break the glass at this stage – you could let choking smoke in. Open the window only if smoke is beginning to build up in the room. Fill your bath with water, and get any remaining towels and bedding soaked ready to cool hotspots. Soak as much as you can of the room – get a mattress against the door, and drench that as a reinforcement for one of your weakest defences. Unless you are very near the ground, don't jump. The result could be serious injury or death. Wait for rescue.

Index